LIPPINCOTT'S
Photo Atlas of
Medication
Administration

Carol Taylor
CSFN, RN, MSN, PhD

Director, Center for Clinical
Bioethics
Assistant Professor, Nursing
Georgetown University
Washington, DC

Carol Lillis
RN, MSN

Interim Dean, Allied Health and Nursing
Department of Nursing
Delaware County Community College
Media, Pennsylvania

Priscilla LeMone
RN, DSN, FAAN

Associate Professor and Director
Undergraduate Program
Sinclair School of Nursing
University of Missouri—Columbia
Columbia, Missouri

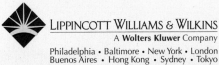

LIPPINCOTT WILLIAMS & WILKINS
A Wolters Kluwer Company

Philadelphia · Baltimore · New York · London
Buenos Aires · Hong Kong · Sydney · Tokyo

Editorial Assistant: Dana Irwin
Senior Production Editor: Sandra Cherrey Scheinin
Senior Production Manager: Helen Ewan
Managing Editor / Production: Erika Kors
Art Director: Carolyn O'Brien
Design Coordinator: Brett MacNaughton
Cover Designer: Christopher Shea
Manufacturing Manager: William Alberti
Indexer: Manjit Sahai
Compositor: Circle Graphics
Printer: Quebecor

9 8 7

ISBN 0-7817-4987-5

Care has been taken to confirm the accuracy of the information presented and to describe generally accepted practices. However, the authors, editors, and publisher are not responsible for errors or omissions or for any consequences from application of the information in this book and make no warranty, express or implied, with respect to the content of the publication.

The authors, editors, and publisher have exerted every effort to ensure that drug selection and dosage set forth in this text are in accordance with the current recommendations and practice at the time of publication. However, in view of ongoing research, changes in government regulations, and the constant flow of information relating to drug therapy and drug reactions, the reader is urged to check the package insert for each drug for any change in indications and dosage and for added warnings and precautions. This is particularly important when the recommended agent is a new or infrequently employed drug.

Some drugs and medical devices presented in this publication have Food and Drug Administration (FDA) clearance for limited use in restricted research settings. It is the responsibility of the health care provider to ascertain the FDA status of each drug or device planned for use in his or her clinical practice.

LWW.com

Contents

Lippincott's Photo Atlas of Medication Administration

Administering Oral Medications

Drugs given orally are intended for absorption in the stomach and small intestine. The oral route is the most commonly used route of administration. It is usually the most convenient and comfortable and is the safest for the patient. Occasionally, a person may unintentionally or intentionally hide a medication in the mouth, or "cheek" it. It is important for the nurse to check that the medication was actually swallowed before recording that it has been taken. After oral administration, drug action has a slower onset and a more prolonged but less potent effect.

There are certain situations in which oral medications would not be administered, such as when the patient has difficulty swallowing, is unconscious, is to receive nothing by mouth, or is vomiting.

Oral medications are available in solid and liquid form. Solid preparations include tablets, capsules, and pills. Some tablets are scored for easy breaking if a partial quantity is needed. *Enteric-coated tablets* are covered with a hard surface that impedes absorption until the tablet has left the stomach.

Absorption takes place in the small intestine because the active ingredient of the drug is irritating to the stomach mucosa. Enteric-coated tablets should not be chewed or crushed.

Liquid preparations include elixirs, spirits, suspensions, and syrups. Some are water-based solutions, and others are alcohol-based solutions. Disposable, calibrated cups are available for the preparation of liquid medications. For patients who find it difficult to take liquids from a cup, the medication can be placed in the mouth directly using a plastic syringe without a needle. The syringe should be placed between the gum and cheek and the liquid given to the patient slowly. This technique, in addition to having the patient in an upright or side-lying position, helps prevent the patient from choking and aspirating the medication.

Certain narcotics that were previously administered parenterally can now also be administered in a lollipop or oral-transmucosal form.

If a label becomes difficult to read or accidentally comes off the container, the container should be returned to the

Box 1
Nursing Responsibilities for Administering Drugs

- Assessment of the patient and clear understanding of why the patient is receiving a particular medication
- Preparing the medication to be administered (ie, checking labels, preparing injections, observing proper asepsis techniques with needles and syringes)
- Accurate dosage calculations
- Administration of the medication (proper injection techniques, aids to help swallowing, topical methods)
- Documentation of medications given
- Monitoring the patient's reaction and evaluating the patient's response
- Educating the patient regarding his or her medications and medication regimen

pharmacy. A medication should never be given from a bottle without a label or with a label that cannot be read with accuracy. Because of the danger of error, unused medications should not be returned to their bottles. Care should be exercised in pouring, to prevent unnecessary loss. Medications should not be transferred from one pharmacy container to another. Many medication bottles now have an identification code number on them. If similar medications were mixed and a patient had a reaction, it would be difficult to identify which drug was responsible. A medication with an unexpected precipitate should not be used, nor should one that has changed color.

Procedure 4 describes the techniques for preparing and administering oral medications.

Special Techniques

Certain drugs that are given orally discolor the teeth or damage the enamel. Such medications are mixed well with water or some other liquid; the patient takes it through a drinking straw, and water is taken after administration. This practice reduces the strength of the drug that comes in contact with the teeth.

Some patients object to the taste of certain medications. The following techniques help disguise or mask the objectionable taste:

- It is sometimes necessary to crush a medication or add it to food so that the patient can swallow it. Some drugs cannot be crushed (eg, enteric-coated and sustained-release capsules). Check with the pharmacist or a pharmacology reference when uncertain about crushing a medication.
- Allow the patient to suck on a small piece of ice for a few minutes before taking the medication. The ice

numbs the taste buds, and the objectionable taste is less discernible.
- Store oily medications in the refrigerator. Cold oil is less aromatic than oil at room temperature.
- Place the medication in a syringe, and place the syringe well back on the tongue, being careful not to trigger the patient's gag reflex. This places the medication on the part of the tongue where there are few taste buds.
- Offer oral hygiene immediately after giving the medication.
- Give the medication with generous amounts of water or other liquids, if permitted, to dilute the taste.

Children

Nurses find administration of medications to infants and children challenging as well as frustrating at times. Children younger than 5 years of age have difficulty swallowing tablets and capsules. Most medications are available in liquid form. Nursing responsibility also includes teaching and preparing family members to administer medications to a child at home. In addition to understanding the medication order and the reason for the medication, the caregiver should be able to demonstrate any special techniques involved in administering the prescribed drugs. Helpful strategies for administering medications to children include the following:

- Use a dropper to give infants or very young children liquid medications while holding them in a sitting or semi-sitting position. Place the medication between the gum and cheek to prevent possible aspiration.
- Crush uncoated tablets or empty a soft capsule and mix the medication with soft foods, such as potatoes or cooked or hot cereal, for patients who are likely to aspirate liquids. Proper absorption may not occur if coated tablets or hard capsules are added to food.
- Explain to the child when a medication has an objectionable taste if the child is old enough to understand. Failing to warn the child is likely to decrease the child's trust in the nurse.
- Care should be taken when selecting the food to be mixed with the medication. The item should not be an essential part of the child's diet, such as formula or the child's favorite food. The child may refuse a food associated with medications.
- Offer the child a flavored ice pop or frozen fruit bar immediately before taking the medication. It numbs the tongue, making the taste of the medication less evident.
- Praise the child for a job well done after he or she swallows the medication.

Older Adults

Techniques for administering medications to older people include the following:

- Allow extra time to administer medications to older patients because their reflexes may be slowed and their understanding of the treatment decreased.
- Older patients may experience some difficulty swallowing medications and may find it easier to take

their medications when crushed or given in liquid form. Swallowing can be initiated by massaging the laryngeal prominence or the area just below the chin prominence. The pressure from the gentle massage creates the desire to swallow. A speech therapist may offer additional suggestions for patients who have difficulty swallowing.

- Reevaluation of the drug dosage is necessary with the older patient. Weight and age should be used as criteria for determining the dosage.
- The nurse should assist the older patient to set up a home medication schedule as a reminder to take medications as scheduled.
- Monitor carefully for adverse effects that may result from the drug regimen. These may be magnified in older individuals.
- Teach patients the names of drugs rather than distinguishing them by color. Manufacturers may vary the colors of generic drugs, and the visual changes associated with aging may make it more difficult to identify medications by their color.

Administering Medications Through an Enteral Feeding Tube

Patients with a gastrointestinal tube (nasogastric, nasointestinal, percutaneous endoscopic gastrostomy [PEG] tube, or J tube) often receive medication through the tube. The following are suggestions for giving medications through the tube:

- Use liquid medications or medications that can be crushed and combined with liquid.
- Bring the liquid medication to room temperature. Cold liquids may cause patient discomfort.
- Remove the clamp from the tube and use the recommended procedure for checking tube placement in the stomach or intestine *before* administering the drug.
- Flush the tube with 15 to 30 mL of water (5 to 10 mL for children) before giving the medication and immediately after giving the medication. Flushing before may warn you if the tube is clogged and helps to maintain tube patency.
- It is best to give medications separately and flush with water between each drug. Some medications may interact with each other or become less effective if mixed with other drugs.
- If the tube is connected to suction, keep it disconnected from the suction and clamped for 20 to 30 minutes after administration of the medication to allow for absorption.
- Disconnect a continuous tube feeding before giving medications, and leave the tube clamped for a short period of time after medication has been given according to agency protocol.
- Document the water intake and liquid medication by tube on the intake and output record. Adjust the amount of water used if the patient is on restricted fluid intake.

Administering Sublingual Medications

Certain drugs, such as sublingual nitroglycerin, are administered *sublingually*; that is, a tablet is placed under the patient's tongue. This area is rich in superficial blood vessels, which allows the drug to be absorbed relatively rapidly into the bloodstream for quick systemic effects. Sublingual medications should not be swallowed but rather are held under the tongue so that complete absorption can occur.

Administering Parenteral Medications

The term *enteral* means within the intestines; parenteral means outside the intestines or alimentary canal. Many people use the term **parenteral** to refer to injection routes only, although technically, the term includes routes for administering agents given by inhalation, those placed on the skin, and most of those placed on the mucous membrane.

Medications may be injected into an artery, the peritoneum, heart tissues, the spinal canal, and bones. Techniques for injecting medications into these areas are discussed in clinical texts. In most instances, physicians are responsible for these procedures, and nurses assist.

Absorption occurs more rapidly with injection than when other routes are used. It is also more nearly complete; therefore, the results are more predictable, and the desired dosage can be determined with greater accuracy. Giving drugs by injection is necessary if the drug is available in no other form. Injections are particularly desirable for patients who are irrational, unconscious, or having gastrointestinal disturbances. The injection of drugs is also used in emergencies because absorption and desired results occur rapidly.

Needles and Syringes

Needles are available in various lengths and gauges with different sizes of bevels. The most commonly used needle lengths vary from $5/16$ inch to 2 inches (0.8 to 5.1 cm). The length of the needle chosen is determined by the route of administration. The gauge is determined by the diameter of the needle. Needle gauges are numbered 18 through 30. As the diameter of the needle increases, the gauge number decreases. An 18-gauge needle is larger than a 30-gauge needle. The bevel of the needle is its sloped edge, designed to make a narrow, slitlike opening that closes quickly.

Syringes are supplied in various sizes. Most syringes are plastic and disposable. Some syringes are supplied with the needle attached, whereas others are not, in which case the nurse selects an appropriate needle.

The nurse chooses the equipment needed for an injection based on the following criteria:

Route of administration: A longer needle is required for an intramuscular injection than for an intradermal or a subcutaneous injection.
Viscosity of the solution: Some medications are more viscous than others and require a large-lumen needle to inject the drug.
Quantity to be administered: The larger the amount of medication to be injected, the greater the capacity of the syringe.

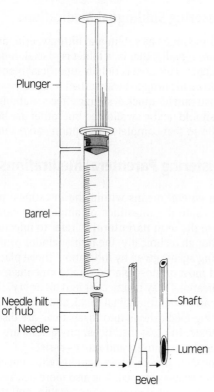

Parts of a needle and syringe.

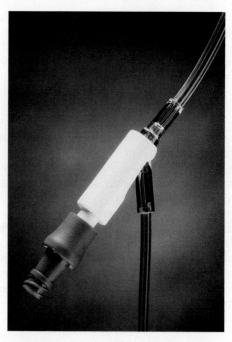

Example of a needleless system. (Courtesy of ICU Medical, Inc., San Clemente, CA.)

Body size: An obese person requires a longer needle to reach muscle tissue than a thin person.

Type of medication: There are special syringes for certain uses. An example is the insulin syringe used to inject insulin. Some medications, such as iron dextran injection (Imferon), are irritating to subcutaneous tissue. Therefore, a longer needle should be used to ensure proper placement of the medication in the muscle tissue.

After use, the needles and syringes are placed in puncture-resistant containers without being recapped. Most needlestick injuries occur during recapping. The one-handed technique is used when a needle must be recapped.

Techniques of surgical asepsis must be strictly followed for parenteral injections to help avoid introducing organisms into the body. The parts of the syringe and needle that must be kept sterile during the procedure of preparing and administering an injection are the inside of the barrel, the part of the plunger that enters the barrel, the tip of the barrel, and the needle, except for the needle's hub.

Surgical asepsis applies to cleaning the skin for an injection. The skin is cleaned with alcohol or povidone-iodine (Betadine) in a circular motion, working from the center of the designated site outward.

Needleless Systems

The risk for accidental needlestick and possible exposure to bloodborne pathogens is reduced significantly with the use of needleless devices or protected needles. These de-

vices prevent needlestick injuries in a variety of ways. Examples include needles that can be sheathed in a plastic guard after the needle is withdrawn from the skin and syringes that have a retractable needle that locks and seals inside the syringe barrel. Needleless systems are also available for intravenous use, including recessed and shielded intravenous needle connectors as well as blunt cannulas that are inserted into special receptor sites on tubing or lock setups. All needleless devices or blunt cannulas are discarded in special containers that are puncture proof, leak proof, clearly labeled, and available at various locations on each healthcare unit.

Preparing Medications for Administration by Injection

Drugs for administration by injection are packaged in several ways. Those that deteriorate in solution are usually dispensed as powders and are reconstituted immediately before injection. If drugs remain stable in solution, they are usually dispensed in ampules, bottles, or vials in an aqueous or oily solution or suspension.

Drugs may be dispensed in single-dose glass ampules, single-dose rubber-capped vials, multidose rubber-capped vials, and prefilled cartridges.

Ampules

An **ampule** is a glass flask that contains a single dose of medication for parenteral administration. There is no way to prevent airborne contamination of any unused portion of medication after the ampule is opened. If all the medication is not used, the remainder must be discarded. Medication is removed from an ampule after its thin neck is

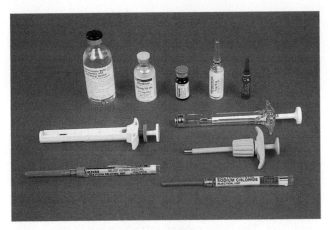

Vials, ampules, prefilled cartridges, and holders.

broken. The ampule can be inverted or placed on a flat surface to draw the solution into the syringe. Care must be taken not to contaminate the needle by touching the rim of the ampule. Procedure 1 shows how to remove medication from an ampule.

Vials

A **vial** is a glass bottle with a self-sealing stopper through which medication is removed. For safety in transporting and storing, the single-dose rubber-capped vial is usually covered with a soft metal cap that can be easily removed. The rubber stopper that is then exposed is the means of entrance into the vial.

Some drugs are dispensed in vials that contain several doses. This means that the nurse can remove several doses from the same container. To facilitate removal of medication, the nurse injects air into the vial. The amount of air is the same as the desired quantity of solution. Procedure 2 details how to remove medication from a vial.

Prefilled Cartridges

Prefilled cartridges provide a single dose of medication. The nurse inserts the cartridge into a reusable holder. Before giving the injection, the nurse checks the dosage in the cartridge and clears the cartridge of excess air. Most prefilled cartridges are overfilled, and the nurse should eject any excess medication to give an exact dose and avoid a medication error. Tubex and Carpuject are two types of prefilled cartridges.

Mixing Medications in One Syringe

Preparation of medications in one syringe depends on how the medication is supplied. When using a single-dose vial and a multidose vial, air is injected into both vials, and the medication in the multidose vial is drawn into the syringe first. This prevents the contents of the multidose vial from being contaminated with the medication in the single-dose vial. The nurse must first ensure that the two drugs are compatible.

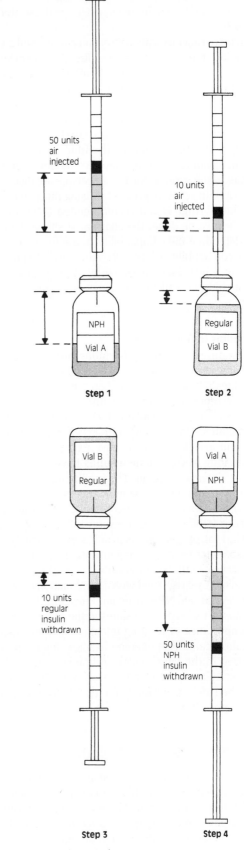

Mixing medications in one syringe.

The steps to follow when preparing medications from two multidose vials in one syringe are illustrated in Procedure 3.

When preparing medications from an ampule and a vial, the medication in the vial is prepared first. The medication in the ampule is drawn up after the medication in the vial.

Nurses must be aware of drug incompatibilities when preparing medications in one syringe. Certain medications, such as diazepam (Valium), are incompatible with other drugs in the same syringe. Other drugs have limited compatibility and should be administered within 15 minutes of preparation. Incompatible drugs may become cloudy or form a precipitate in the syringe. Such medications are discarded and reprepared in separate syringes. Mixing more than two drugs in one syringe is not recommended (McConnell, 1998b). If it must be done, the pharmacist should be contacted to determine the compatibility of the three drugs as well as the compatibility of their pH values and the preservatives that may be present in each drug. A drug compatibility table should be available to nurses who are preparing medications.

Mixing Insulins in One Syringe

Insulin, a naturally occurring hormone produced by the islets of Langerhans in the pancreas, enables cells to use carbohydrates. Patients with diabetes mellitus produce no insulin or produce insulin in insufficient amounts. Several types of insulin are available for use by patients with diabetes mellitus. Insulins vary in their onset and duration of action and are classified as short acting, intermediate acting, and long acting. Some insulins have a modifying protein that slows absorption. The modifying proteins are globin and protamine (NPH, globin zinc, protamine zinc).

Insulin dosages are calculated in units. The scale commonly used is U100, which is based on 100 units of insulin contained in 1 mL of solution. An insulin syringe is calibrated in units also. Before administering insulin, the nurse should check the dosage with the physician's orders. Many cases of diabetes mellitus are regulated with a combination of two insulins (eg, regular and NPH insulins). Procedure 3 gives the steps for mixing two types of insulins in the same syringe.

The importance of rotating injection sites for insulin administration cannot be overemphasized. Injection sites are discussed in the later section, Administering Medications Subcutaneously. A 10-mL vial of unrefrigerated insulin may be safely used for 1 month if stored in a cool place (Fleming, 1999).

Reconstituting Powdered Medications

Occasionally, a drug may be supplied as a powder in a vial. A liquid, or *diluent*, must be added to the powder before it is administered as a solution. The technique of adding a diluent to a powdered drug is called *reconstitution*. Information needed for reconstitution and dosage calculation is usually located on the vial label. Additional sources of information about reconstitution of medications are package inserts and the pharmacist.

Administering Medications Intradermally

The intradermal route has the longest absorption time of all parenteral routes. For this reason, intradermal injections are used for diagnostic purposes, such as the tuberculin test and tests to determine sensitivity to various substances. The advantage of the intradermal route for these tests is that the body's reaction to substances is easily visible, and degrees of reaction are discernible by comparative study.

Intradermal injections are placed just below the epidermis. Sites commonly used are the inner surface of the forearm, the dorsal aspect of the upper arm, and the upper back. Equipment used for an intradermal injection include a tuberculin syringe calibrated in tenths and hundredths of a milliliter. The dosage given intradermally is small, usually less than 0.5 mL. A $\frac{1}{4}$- to $\frac{1}{2}$-inch (0.6 to 1.3 cm), 26- or 27-gauge needle is used. Procedure 5 shows how to administer an intradermal injection.

Administering Medications Subcutaneously

Subcutaneous tissue lies between the epidermis and the muscle. Because there is subcutaneous tissue all over the body, various sites are used for **subcutaneous injections**. These sites are the outer aspect of the upper arm, the abdomen (from below the costal margin to the iliac crests), anterior aspects of the thigh, upper back, and the upper ventral or dorsogluteal area. This route is used to administer insulin, heparin, and certain immunizations.

Equipment used for a subcutaneous injection depends on the medication to be given. For instance, insulin is prepared with an insulin syringe. Heparin is prepared with a tuberculin syringe or supplied in a prefilled cartridge. A $\frac{5}{16}$- to 1-inch, 25- to 30-gauge needle is used for this route. Ordinarily, no more than 1 mL of solution is given subcutaneously. Giving larger amounts adds to the patient's discomfort and may predispose to poor absorption.

The skin is cleaned for a subcutaneous injection in the same manner as for an intradermal injection. Recent research has questioned the need to clean the skin with an alcohol prep before an insulin injection. The combination of a small-gauge needle that limits the number of bacteria that can pass through it and bacteriostatic additives in insulin preparations makes skin preparation before an insulin injection unnecessary. However, this cleansing is still commonly performed (Fleming, 1999).

The nurse chooses the angle of needle insertion based on the amount of subcutaneous tissue present and the length of the needle. In most cases, a $\frac{5}{8}$-inch needle is inserted at a 45-degree angle and a $\frac{1}{2}$-inch needle is inserted at a 90-degree angle. The patient's size may also determine the angle of needle insertion. For a thin patient, it is best to bunch the skin to create a skin fold and insert the needle at a 45-degree angle. The risk for injecting a medication intramuscularly is lower for a heavier person, and a 90-degree angle may be used. Because the needle frequently used now for insulin injections is thinner (30 gauge) and shorter ($\frac{5}{16}$ inch), the angle of needle insertion is less important.

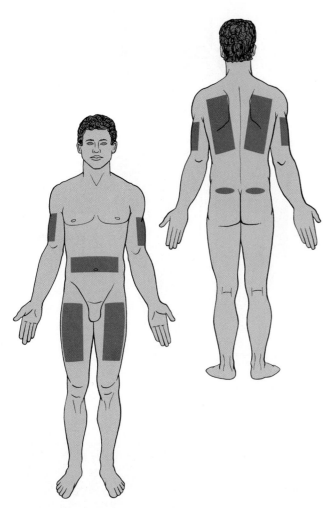

Sites on the body where subcutaneous injections can be given.

It is unlikely, even in a thin person, that this smaller needle will reach muscle tissue.

Heparin is also administered subcutaneously; the abdomen is the most commonly used site. The area two inches around the umbilicus and the belt line must be avoided. Manufacturer's directions for subcutaneous administration of low-molecular-weight heparin preparations (eg, Lovenox) include specific instructions to pinch the tissue gently and insert the needle at a 90-degree angle into a fat pad on either side of the abdomen. Aspiration or pulling back on the plunger is not recommended with administration of heparin because this action can result in hematoma formation. Aspiration after an insulin injection is also unnecessary and has not proved a reliable indicator of needle placement. For a subcutaneous injection, the site is gently massaged after the medication has been given, except in the case of heparin and insulin because massaging the site can increase the rate of absorption of these agents.

It is necessary to rotate sites or areas for injection if the patient is to receive frequent injections. This helps to prevent buildup of fibrous tissue and permits complete absorption of the medication. It is recommended that patients administering their own insulin use the same area of the body at the same time every day to ensure more consistent

absorption (Fleming, 1999). Insulin is absorbed most quickly in the abdomen, followed by the arms, thighs, and buttocks. For instance, every morning the patient uses the abdomen for insulin injection and every evening before dinner, the patient injects the insulin into the arms or thighs. In each case, the injections should be given an inch away from the previous injection site so that the same area will not be used again in the same month. A small spot bandage or piece of tape can be used to mark the first injection site, with subsequent injections rotated in a circle around that site. After this area has been used, an adjacent site, an inch away, can be selected, using the same rotation format. A marked diagram incorporated into the patient's plan of care is also helpful for noting alternative sites. It is futile to rely on memory. Not even the patient can always recall the site of the previous injection. The site of administration is recorded in the patient's record. Procedure 6 shows the procedure for administering medications subcutaneously. Techniques for reducing discomfort in subcutaneous administrations are listed after the discussion Administering Medications Intramuscularly.

Administering Medications Intramuscularly

The intramuscular route is often used for drugs that are irritating because there are few nerve endings in deep muscle tissue. If a sore or inflamed muscle is entered, however, the muscle may act as a trigger area, and severe referred pain often results. It is best to palpate a muscle before injection. A site should be selected that does not feel tender to the patient and where the tissue does not contract and become firm and tense.

Absorption occurs as in subcutaneous administration but more rapidly because of the greater vascularity of muscle tissue. The amount of 4 mL is considered the maximum to be given in one site for an adult with well-developed muscles, although the patient's size and the site used (eg, deltoid muscle) may necessitate that a smaller amount is injected (Beyea & Nicoll, 1996).

Intramuscular Injection Sites

An important point in the administration of an **intramuscular injection** is the selection of a safe site away from large nerves, bones, and blood vessels. When care is not taken, common complications include abscesses, necrosis and skin slough, nerve injuries, lingering pain, and periostitis (inflammation of the membrane covering a bone).

The sites for injecting intramuscular medications should be rotated when therapy requires repeated injections. The sites described in this chapter may all be used on a rotating basis. Whatever pattern of rotating sites is used, a description of it should appear in the patient's plan of nursing care.

Ventrogluteal Site

The ventrogluteal site involves the gluteus medius and gluteus minimus muscles in the hip area. The ventrogluteal site is recommended for both adults and children older than 7 months of age as a safe site for most intramuscular injections. There are no large nerves or blood vessels in the

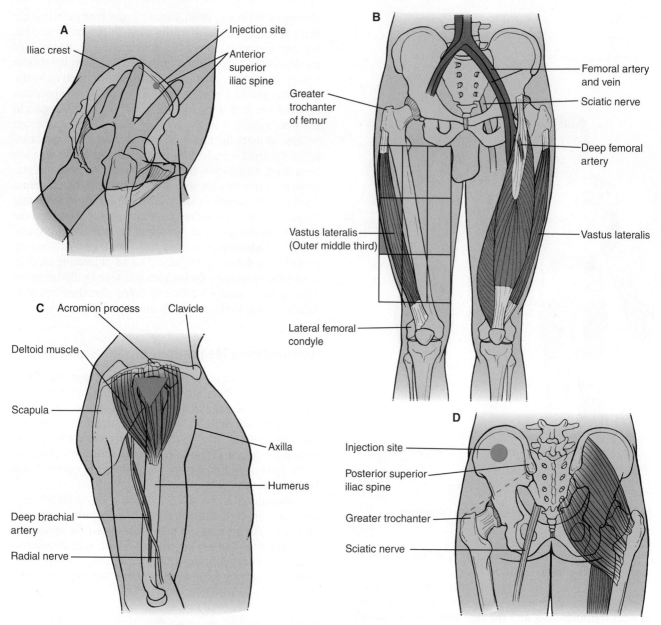

Sites for intramuscular injections. Descriptions for locating the sites are given in the text. (**A**) The *ventrogluteal site* is located by placing the palm on the greater trochanter and the index finger toward the anterosuperior iliac spine. (**B**) The *vastus lateralis site* is identified by dividing the thigh into thirds, horizontally and vertically. (**C**) The *deltoid muscle site* is located by palpating the lower edge of the acromion process. (**D**) The *dorsogluteal site* is lateral and slightly superior to the midpoint of a line drawn from the trochanter to the posterior superior iliac spine.

injection area, the site is removed from bone tissue, the area is clean because fecal contamination is rare at this site, and the patient can be on the back, abdomen, or side for the injection. To relax the gluteal muscle, the patient may flex the knees while lying on the back, point the toes inward while lying in the prone position, and flex the upper leg in front of the lower leg in the side-lying position. Although any of the three positions just described may be used when injecting the ventrogluteal site, nurses increasingly prefer the side-lying position.

To locate the ventrogluteal site, the nurse places the palm over the greater trochanter, with the fingers facing the patient's head. The right hand is used for the patient's left hip, or the left hand for the right hip, to identify landmarks. The index finger is placed on the anterosuperior iliac spine, and the middle finger extends dorsally, palpating the crest of the ileum. A triangle is formed. The injection is made in the center of the triangle.

Vastus Lateralis Site

The vastus lateralis muscle is recommended frequently for the injection of medications if the ventrogluteal site cannot be used. It is a thick muscle, and there is little or no danger of serious injury. There are no large nerves or vessels in proximity, and it does not cover a joint. The muscle covers the anterolateral aspect of the thigh. It is bounded by the midanterior thigh on the front of the leg and the midlateral thigh on the side. The thigh is divided into thirds horizontally and vertically. The injection is given in the *outer middle* third. This space provides a large number of injection sites. The vastus lateralis site is particularly desirable for infants and children, whose gluteal muscles are poorly developed.

Deltoid Muscle Site

The deltoid muscle is located in the lateral aspect of the upper arm. It is not often used because it is a small muscle and is not capable of absorbing large amounts of solution. Damage to the radial nerve and artery is a risk of the deltoid site. Intramuscular injections into the deltoid muscle should be limited to 1 mL of solution and used only for adults. The deltoid muscle is not developed enough in infants and children to absorb medication adequately.

The deltoid muscle can be located by palpating the lower edge of the acromion process. A triangle is formed at the midpoint in line with the axilla on the lateral aspect of the upper arm. Hepatitis B virus vaccine is one medication that should be given in the deltoid muscle in adults to induce adequate levels of the antibody.

Dorsogluteal Site

The dorsogluteal site, located in the buttock, has been a common site for administering intramuscular injections. Because of the potential for accidental injury to the sciatic nerve and the presence of major blood vessels and bone mass near the site, the dorsogluteal muscle is not considered an optimal site. The posterosuperior iliac spine and the greater trochanter represent the anatomic landmarks. An imaginary line is drawn between the posterosuperior iliac spine and the greater trochanter. The injection site is lateral and slightly superior to the midpoint of the line. The gluteal muscles are developed by walking; therefore, the dorsogluteal site is not to be used for children younger than 3 years of age because their gluteal muscles are too small.

Good visualization of the entire area and careful mapping are necessary to locate the proper site. This necessitates adequate exposure by lowering the undergarments. Merely raising one side of underclothing permits only a partial visualization of the area. It is recommended that the patient be in a prone position with the toes pointed inward, or in the side-lying position with the upper knee flexed and the upper leg in front of the lower leg. These positions help to promote maximum muscle relaxation and, therefore, minimum discomfort. When the patient is in a standing position, the gluteus muscle usually is tense, and then this site should not be used.

Intramuscular Injection Procedure

No more than 4 mL should be injected into a single injection site for an adult with well-developed muscles. The less developed muscles of children and elderly people limit the intramuscular injection to 1 to 2 mL. Equipment commonly used for an intramuscular injection includes a 1½-inch (3.8 cm), 21- to 23-gauge needle. The length of the needle should be selected with care for any intramuscular injection. Prepackaged, loaded syringes usually have a needle that is

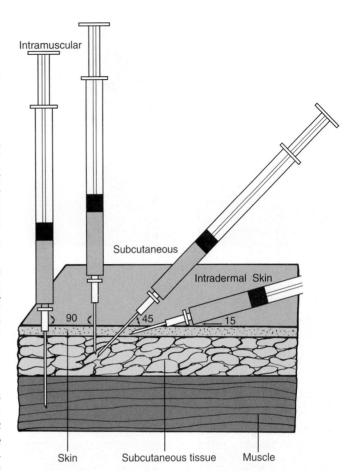

Comparison of the angles of insertion for intramuscular, subcutaneous, and intradermal injections.

1 inch long. If there is any question about whether the belly of the target muscle can be reached, the medication should be transferred to another syringe with the appropriate needle size. A short needle does not minimize discomfort, and a longer one does not increase discomfort. The characteristics of the patient's anatomy should dictate the needle length chosen. The most important consideration is to use a needle with a tip that will reach deep into the muscle.

The addition of an air bubble to the syringe is unnecessary and a potentially dangerous procedure that could result in an overdose of medication. Disposable syringes are calibrated to deliver a correct dose without the use of an air bubble (Beyea & Nicoll, 1996). The technique for administering an intramuscular injection is outlined in Procedure 7.

Z-Track Technique

Any intramuscular injection may be given using the **Z-track** technique. Beyea & Nicoll (1996) state that Z-track is the safest and most comfortable technique for giving any intramuscular injection. This prevents seepage of the medication into the needle track and reduces the pain and discomfort, particularly for patients receiving injections over an extended period. In the Z-track technique, a clean needle is attached to the syringe after the syringe is filled with the medication to prevent the injection of any residual medication on the needle into superficial tissues. The

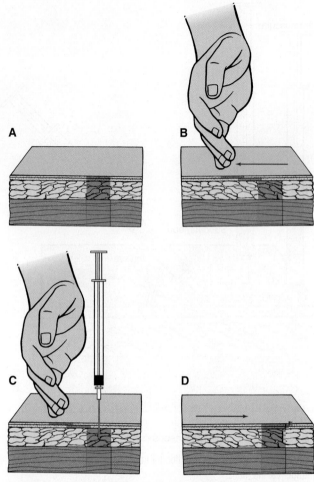

The Z-track or zigzag technique is recommended for intramuscular injections. (**A**) Normal skin and tissues. (**B**) Moving the skin to one side. (**C**) Needle is inserted at a 90-degree angle, and needle is aspirated for blood. (**D**) Once the needle is withdrawn, displaced tissue is allowed to return to its normal position, preventing the solution from escaping from the muscle tissue.

needle should be a minimum of 1½ inches (3.8 cm) long. The ventrogluteal, vastus lateralis, or dorsogluteal site can be used for this procedure. The skin is pulled down or to one side about 1 inch (2.5 cm), and held in this position with the left hand for a right-handed person. The needle is inserted and aspirated carefully to detect the presence of blood. The medication is injected slowly, the needle is then steadily withdrawn, and the displaced tissue is released and allowed to return to its normal position.

Massage of the site is not recommended because it may cause irritation by forcing the medication to leak back into the needle track, but gentle pressure may be applied with a dry sponge.

Reducing Discomfort in Subcutaneous and Intramuscular Administrations

The following are recommended techniques to help reduce discomfort when injecting medications subcutaneously or intramuscularly:

- Select a needle of the smallest gauge that is appropriate for the site and solution to be injected, and select the correct needle length.
- Be sure the needle is free of medication that may irritate superficial tissues as the needle is inserted. Recommended procedure is to use two needles—one to remove the medication from the vial or ampule and a second one to inject the medication. If medication is in a prefilled syringe with a nonremovable needle and has dripped back on the needle during preparation, gently tap the barrel to remove the excess solution.
- Use the Z-track technique for intramuscular injections to prevent leakage of medication into the needle track, thus minimizing the patient's discomfort.
- Inject the medication into relaxed muscles. There is more pressure and discomfort when the medication is injected into a contracted muscle.
- Do not inject areas that feel hard on palpation or tender to the patient.
- Insert the needle with a dartlike motion without hesitation, and remove it quickly at the same angle at which it was inserted. These techniques help to reduce discomfort and tissue irritation.
- Do not administer more solution in one injection than is recommended for the site. Injecting more solution creates excess pressure in the area and increases discomfort.
- Inject the solution slowly so that it may be dispersed more easily into the surrounding tissue (10 seconds per 1 mL).
- Apply gentle pressure after injection, unless this technique is contraindicated.
- Allow the patient who is fearful of injections to talk about his or her fears. Answer the patient's questions truthfully, and explain the nature and purpose of the injection. Taking the time to offer support often allays fears that ordinarily add to the discomfort of the procedure for the patient.
- Rotate the sites when the patient is to receive repeated injections. Injections in the same site may cause undue discomfort, irritation, or abscesses in tissues.

Administering Medications Intravenously

Medications administered intravenously have an immediate effect. The **intravenous route** is the most dangerous route of administration. Because the drug is placed directly into the bloodstream, it cannot be recalled, nor can its actions be slowed. Intravenous administration is the route used in most emergency situations when immediate absorption is required. There also are many nonemergency clinical situations in which drugs are administered intravenously. Patient-controlled analgesia allows the patient to control administration of an intravenous analgesic for pain management. Procedure 10 describes the basic technique for administering an intravenous infusion.

There are several ways to administer medications intravenously. Medications may be added to the patient's infusion solution. The recommended procedure is for the pharmacist to add the prescribed drug to a large volume of intravenous solution, but sometimes the drug is added in the nursing unit, in which case sterile technique must be maintained. Steps for adding medications to intravenous solutions are given in Procedure 15.

When medication is administered by *continuous infusion*, the patient receives it slowly and over a long period. Although sometimes this can be an advantage when it is desirable to give the medication slowly, it is a disadvantage when the patient needs to receive the drug more quickly. Also, if for some reason all of the solution cannot be infused, the patient will not receive the prescribed amount of the medication. The patient receiving medication by a continuous intravenous infusion should be checked for possible adverse effects at least every hour.

A medication can be administered as an intravenous *bolus* or push. This involves a single injection of a concentrated solution administered directly into an intravenous line (Procedure 16).

Medications can be administered by *intermittent intravenous infusion*. The drug is mixed with a small amount of the intravenous solution, such as 50 to 100 mL, and administered over a short period at the prescribed interval, for example, every 4 hours. As mentioned earlier, needleless devices are recommended by the Centers for Disease Control and Prevention and the Occupational Safety and Health Administration, and they effectively prevent needlesticks and provide access to the primary venous line. Either blunt-ended cannulas or recessed connection ports may be used. A patient with an intravenous line in place can receive the solution containing the medication by way of a piggyback setup, a volume-control administration set (eg, Pediatrol or Volutrol), or a miniinfusion pump. The intravenous *piggyback* delivery system requires the intermittent or additive solution to be placed higher than the primary solution container. An extension hook provided by the manufacturer provides for easy lowering of the main intravenous container. The port on the primary intravenous line has a back-check valve that automatically stops the flow of the primary solution, allowing the secondary or piggyback solution to flow when connected. A *tandem* delivery setup is similar, except that both solutions remain at the same height and there is no back-check valve at the secondary port on the primary line. This type of setup is used infrequently because the solution from the primary intravenous line will back up into the tandem line if this intermittent infusion is not clamped immediately after it is infused. Because manufacturer's designs vary, nurses are advised to check the directions carefully for the systems used in their agency. The nurse is responsible for calculating and manually adjusting the flow rate of the intravenous intermittent infusion or regulating the infusion with an infusion pump or controller. Intravenous administration of medications using additive sets is explained in Procedure 17.

Medications can also be placed in a controlled-volume administration set for intermittent intravenous infusion. The medication is diluted with a small amount of solution and administered through the patient's intravenous line

(see Procedure 17). This type of equipment is also used for infusing solutions into children and older patients when the volume of fluid infused must be carefully monitored.

The minisyringe pump for intermittent infusion is battery operated and allows medication mixed in a syringe to be connected to the primary line and delivered by mechanical pressure applied to the syringe plunger (see Procedure 17).

A *heparin or saline lock*, or intermittent venous access device, is used for patients who require intermittent intravenous medication but not a continuous intravenous infusion. This device consists of a needle or catheter connected to a short length of tubing capped with a sealed injection port. An intravenous lock is shown in Procedure 18. After the needle is in place in the patient's vein, the needle and tubing are anchored to the patient's arm so that the needle remains in place until the patient no longer requires the repeated medication intravenously.

An intravenous lock allows the patient more freedom than a continuous intravenous infusion. The patient is connected to the intravenous line when it is time to receive the medication and disconnected when the medication is completed. A saline flush rather than a heparin flush is used in many agencies to maintain patency of the heparin lock. Using saline eliminates any possible systemic effects on coagulation or drug incompatibility that may occur when a heparin solution is used. The intermittent infusion is not started until the nurse confirms intravenous placement. The heparin lock is flushed after the infusion is completed to clear the vein of any medication and to prevent clot formation in the needle. The procedure for flushing an intravenous lock with saline is discussed in Procedure 18. If infiltration or phlebitis occurs, the lock is removed and replaced in a new site.

In addition to a peripheral intravenous line, intermittent intravenous medication may be administered through a centrally placed line into the subclavian or internal jugular veins or through peripherally inserted central catheters. Medications are prepared under laminar flow in a sterile environment if they are to be administered through a central intravenous line, such as a Hickman catheter. Laminar flow is a special technique that helps regulate air flow to prevent bacterial contamination and collection of hazardous chemical fumes. Aseptic technique is observed when the nurse administers medications through a central intravenous line. All connections are cleaned with povidone-iodine or an antiseptic agent.

Administering Topical Medications

When a drug is applied directly to a body site, it is called a **topical application**. Topical applications are usually intended for direct action at a particular site, although some systemic effect may also occur. The action depends on the type of tissue and the nature of the agent.

If the site of application is readily accessible, such as the skin, an agent can easily be placed on it. If it is a cavity, such as the nose, or is enclosed, such as the eye, it is necessary to use a mechanical applicator for introducing the drug.

Skin Applications

The skin is a mechanical and chemical barrier that protects the underlying tissues. It is a sense organ, having receptors that respond to touch, pain, pressure, and temperature. The skin helps in excretion, in regulating body temperature, and in storing essentials to the body, such as water, salts, and glucose.

When a drug is incorporated in an agent, such as an ointment, and rubbed into the skin for absorption, the procedure is referred to as an *inunction*. On normal skin, drugs are absorbed into the lining of the sebaceous glands. Absorption is hindered because of the protective outer layer of the skin, which makes penetration difficult, and because of the fatty substances that protect the lining of the glands. Absorption can be enhanced by cleaning the skin well with soap or detergent and water before administration and then rubbing the medicated preparation into the skin. Absorption can also be improved by using a drug mixed in an ointment or added to a liniment that will mix with the fat in the gland lining. When indicated, local heat applied to the application area can improve blood circulation and promote absorption. The following are typical preparations applied to skin areas:

Powders are used to promote drying of the skin and prevent friction on the skin. Use caution when applying to prevent inhalation of the powder.

Ointments provide prolonged contact of a medication with the skin and soften the skin. They are usually thoroughly massaged into intact skin.

Creams and oils lubricate and soften the skin and prevent drying of the skin. The preparation should be warmed in the hands or fingers if a large part of the body is to be covered, to prevent chilling.

Lotions protect and soothe the skin. Shake lotions thoroughly before using and apply with cotton balls or gauze.

The *transdermal* route is being used more frequently to deliver medication. This involves application of a disk or patch to the skin that contains medication intended for daily use or for longer intervals. Despite a slow onset of action, transdermal drug patches maintain consistent serum drug levels (see Box 2).

Box 2
Guidelines for Nursing Care
Applying Transdermal Patches

- Wear gloves when applying or removing patches. Handwashing is also a necessity.
- Remove the old patch before applying the new one. The physician may order a specific time for removal of the patch that may not coincide with the application time.
- Dispose of old patches carefully. Keep out of the reach of children and away from pets.
- Follow directions and use the patch as prescribed. Remove the patch from its protective covering and then remove the clear plastic covering without touching the adhesive. Apply the patch and use the palm to press firmly for about 10 seconds.
- Rotate application sites.
- Apply the patch at the same time of the day and write the date and time on the patch. Document application on the MAR.
- Monitor the patient's response carefully. Be alert for adverse effects specific to the medication applied.
- Check for dislodgment of the patch if the patient is active. Read information about the patch or consult with the pharmacist to determine reapplication schedule and procedure.
- Assess for any skin irritation. If necessary, remove the patch, wash the area carefully with soap and water, and allow skin to air dry.
- Aluminum backing on a patch necessitates precautions if defibrillation is required. Burns and smoke may result.

Adapted from McConnell, E. (1997). Using transdermal medication patches. *Nursing, 27*(7), 18.

Eye Instillations and Irrigations

The receptors for the sense of sight are located in the eye. The outer layer of the eyeball is called the *sclera*. The cornea is the transparent part of the sclera in front of the eyeball. The sclera is fibrous and tough, but the cornea is easily injured by trauma. For this reason, applications to the eye seldom are placed directly onto the eyeball.

Because direct application cannot be made onto the sensitive cornea, applications intended to act on the eye or the lids are placed onto, or instilled or irrigated into, the lower conjunctival sac.

The eye is a delicate organ, highly susceptible to infection and injury. Although the eye is never free of microorganisms, the secretions of the conjunctiva have a protective action against many pathogens. For maximum safety for the patient, the equipment, solutions, and ointments introduced into the conjunctival sac should be sterile. If this is not possible, the most careful guidelines for medical asepsis should be followed.

Eyedrops

Instillation of eyedrops is performed for their local effects, such as for pupil dilation or constriction when examining the eye, for treating an infection, or to aid in controlling intraocular pressure for patients with glaucoma. The type and amount of solution depend on the purpose of the instillation. See the accompanying Box 3, Instilling Eyedrops, for a description of techniques to expose the lower conjunctival sac and instill eyedrops.

Box 3
Guidelines for Nursing Care

Instilling Eyedrops

- Offer the patient paper tissues to remove solution and tears that may spill from the eye during the procedure.
- Wash hands before putting on gloves.
- Clean the eyelids and eyelashes of any drainage with cotton balls or gauze pledgets moistened with normal saline solution because debris can be carried into the eye when the conjunctival sac is exposed. Use each cotton ball for only one stroke, moving from the inner toward the outer canthus to prevent carrying debris to the lacrimal ducts.
- Tilt the patient's head back slightly if sitting, or place the patient's head over a pillow if lying down. The head may be turned slightly to the affected side to prevent solution or tears from flowing toward the opposite eye.
- Invert the monodrip plastic container that is commonly used to instill eyedrops.
- Have the patient look up while focusing on something on the ceiling.

- Place the thumb or two fingers near the margin of the lower eyelid immediately below the eyelashes, and exert pressure downward over the bony prominence of the cheek. The lower conjunctival sac is exposed as the lower lid is pulled down.
- Hold the dropper close to the eye, but avoid touching the eyelids or lashes, which may startle the patient and cause blinking. Also, avoid touching the eyeball with the dropper because this could easily injure the eye.
- Squeeze the container and allow the prescribed number of drops to fall in the lower conjunctival sac. Do not allow drops to fall onto the cornea because of the danger of injuring it and the unpleasant sensation it causes the patient.
- Release the lower lid after the eyedrops are instilled. Ask the patient to close the eyes gently.
- Apply gentle pressure over the inner canthus to prevent the eyedrops from flowing into the tear duct. This minimizes the risk of systemic effects from the medication.
- Instruct patient not to rub the affected eye.

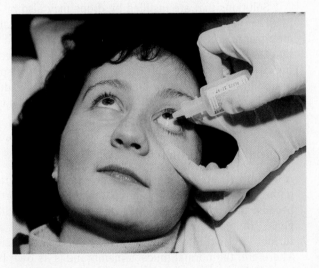

With the lower lid pulled down, the nurse prepares to administer the eyedrops on the lower conjunctival sac.

Ointments

Various types of medication in an ointment form may be prescribed for the eye. These ointments are usually used for a local infection or irritation. Eye ointments are dispensed in a tube. A small amount of ointment is distributed along the exposed lower conjunctival sac after the eyelids and eyelashes have been cleansed. About $\frac{1}{2}$ inch of ointment is squeezed from the tube along the exposed sac. After the application, the eyes should be closed. The warmth helps to liquefy the ointment. Also, the patient should be instructed to move the eye because this helps to spread ointment under the lids and over the surface of the eyeball.

Eye Irrigation

An eye *irrigation* is performed to remove secretions or foreign bodies or to cleanse and soothe the eye. In an emergency, eye irrigation can be used to remove chemicals that may burn the eye. Copious amounts of tap water should be used to remove chemicals such as acid. The irrigation should continue for at least 15 minutes, and then professional help should be sought.

The techniques for administering an eye irrigation are described in Procedure 8.

Eye Medication Disks

An eye medication disk is flexible, resembles a contact lens, and contains medication that is gradually released into the conjunctival sac. It can remain in place for up to a week before being removed and discarded. When properly placed, the disk is completely covered by the lower eyelid, allowing the patient to wear contact lenses, swim, and sleep with the disk in place. Gloves should be worn when applying and removing the disk. Additional nursing guidelines for inserting and removing an intraocular disk include the following:

- Position the disk with the convex side adhering to your fingertip.
- Ask the patient to look up, and use the other hand to pull the patient's lower eyelid down gently.
- Place the disk in the conjunctival sac and lift the lower eyelid up and over the disk. *If properly positioned, the disk should not be visible at this time.*
- For removal, expose the disk by pulling down on the patient's lower eyelid.
- Use the forefinger and thumb of the other hand to gently pinch the disk and lift it out of the patient's eye.

These medication disks are usually applied at bedtime because they initially cause blurring of vision.

Ear Instillations and Irrigations

The ear contains the receptors for hearing and for equilibrium. It consists of the external ear, the middle ear, and the inner ear. The external ear consists of the auricle or pinna and the exterior auditory canal. The auditory canal serves as a passageway for sound waves. Drugs or irrigations are instilled into the auditory canal for their local effect. They are used to soften wax, relieve pain, apply local anesthesia, destroy organisms, or destroy an insect lodged in the canal, which can cause almost intolerable discomfort.

The tympanic membrane separates the external ear from the middle ear. Normally, it is intact and closes the entrance to the middle ear completely. If it is ruptured or has been opened by surgical intervention, the middle ear and the inner ear have a direct passage to the external ear. When this occurs, instillations and irrigations should be performed with the greatest of care to prevent forcing materials from the outer ear into the middle ear and the inner ear. Sterile technique is used to prevent infection.

Ear Drops

The techniques listed in the accompanying Box 4, Instilling Ear Drops, are recommended to place drops in the external auditory canal.

Ear Irrigations

Irrigations of the external auditory canal are ordinarily for cleaning purposes or for applying heat to the area. Typically, normal saline solution is used, although an antiseptic solution may be indicated for local action. An irrigation syringe is used in most instances. An irrigating container with tubing and an ear tip may also be used, especially if the purpose of the irrigation is to apply heat to the area. The techniques for administering an irrigation of the external auditory canal are described in Procedure 9.

Nasal Instillations

Besides serving as the olfactory organ, the nose functions as an airway to the lower respiratory tract and protects the tract by cleaning and warming the air taken in by inspiration. Cilia project on most of the surfaces of the nasal mucous membrane and help remove particles of dirt and dust from the inspired air. The nose also serves as a resonator when speaking and singing.

Nasal instillations are used to treat sinus infections and nasal congestion. Medications with a systemic effect, such as vasopressin, may also be prepared as a nasal instillation. The nose is normally not a sterile cavity, but because of its connection with the sinuses, medical asepsis should be carefully observed when using nasal instillations. See the accompanying Box 5, Instilling Nose Drops, for recommended techniques to instill nose drops.

Solutions that are instilled by drops may also be applied to the nasal mucous membrane in a spray. A small atomizer is used. The end of the nose is held up, and the tip of the nozzle is placed just inside the nares and directed backward. Only sufficient force is used to bring the spray into contact with the membrane. Too much force may drive the solution and contamination into the sinuses and eustachian tubes.

Vaginal Applications

A healthy vagina contains few pathogens but many nonpathogenic organisms. The nonpathogens are important because they protect the vagina from the invasion of pathogens. The normal secretions in the vagina are acidic and further serve to protect the vagina from microbial invasion. Therefore, the normal mucous membrane is its own best protection.

Creams can be applied intravaginally, using a narrow, tubular applicator with an attached plunger. Suppositories that melt when exposed to body heat are also administered by vaginal insertion. Suppositories should be refrigerated for storage.

The patient should be asked to void before inserting the medication. The patient is positioned lying on her back with the knees flexed. Privacy should be maintained with draping. Adequate light should be available to visualize the vaginal opening (see the accompanying Box 6, Inserting Vaginal Suppository or Cream).

Box 4
Guidelines for Nursing Care

Instilling Ear Drops

- Warm the solution to be instilled to body temperature to minimize discomfort for the patient.
- Clean the external ear of drainage with cotton balls moistened with normal saline solution, as necessary. (Disposable gloves should be worn if drainage is present.)
- Place the patient on the unaffected side in bed, or if ambulatory, have the patient sit with the head well tilted to the side so that the affected ear is uppermost. This positioning prevents the drops from escaping from the ear.
- Draw up the amount of solution needed in the dropper. Excess medication should not be returned to a stock bottle. A monodrip plastic container may also be used.
- Straighten the auditory canal by pulling the cartilaginous portion of the pinna up and back in an adult and down and back in an infant or a child under age 3 years, and straight back for a school-aged child. Pulling on the pinna as described helps to straighten the canal properly for ear instillation.
- Hold the dropper in the ear with its tip above the auditory canal. For an infant or an irrational or restless patient, protect the dropper with a piece of soft tubing to help prevent injury to the ear.
- Allow the drops to fall on the side of the canal. It is uncomfortable for the patient if drops fall directly onto the tympanic membrane.
- Release the pinna after instilling the drops, and have the patient maintain the position to prevent the escape of the medication.
- Gently press on the tragus a few times to help move the medication from the canal toward the tympanic membrane.
- If ordered, loosely insert a cotton ball to prevent medication from leaking out.
- Wait 5 minutes before instilling drops in the second ear, if ordered.

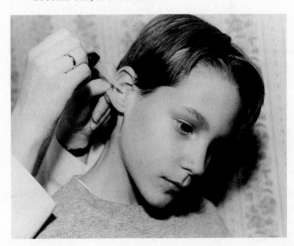

Adult   School-aged child

Rectal Instillations

Rectal suppositories are used primarily for their local action, such as laxatives and fecal softeners. Systemic effects are also achieved with rectal suppositories. Acetaminophen suppositories are used for an antipyretic effect, and many antiemetics are available in suppository form to relieve nausea and vomiting.

Clean disposable gloves should be used to prevent contamination with feces and microorganisms. After the suppository is inserted, the patient should remain in that position for 5 minutes. If the suppository is for laxative purposes, it must remain in position for 35 to 45 minutes or until the patient feels the urge to defecate.

Administering Medications by Inhalation

The lungs are richly supplied with blood and have a large surface area. These characteristics allow drugs to be absorbed easily from the lower respiratory tract. The smaller the particles of inhaled medication, the lower in the respiratory tract the medication tends to travel. A disadvantage of using this route is that the drug dosage is difficult to establish.

Box 5
Guidelines for Nursing Care

Instilling Nose Drops

- Provide the patient with paper tissues and ask that the patient blow his or her nose before instilling the nose drops.
- Have the patient sit up with head tilted well back. Or, if the patient is lying down, tilt the head back over a pillow. These positions allow the solution to flow well back into the nares.
- Draw sufficient solution into the dropper for both nares. Excess solution should not be returned to a stock bottle.
- Hold up the tip of the nose and place the dropper just inside the nares about one third of an inch. Instill the prescribed number of drops in one naris and then into the other. Protect the dropper with a piece of soft tubing when the patient is an infant or young child.
- Avoid touching the nares with the dropper because it may cause the patient to sneeze.
- Have the patient remain in position with the head tilted back for a few minutes to prevent the escape of the solution.

Drugs classified as bronchodilators and decongestants commonly are administered by **inhalation**. They act to decrease resistance to air flow by enlarging air passageways. Decongestants are local vasoconstrictors. Bronchodilators promote relaxation of musculature in the tracheobronchial tree. The relaxed passages produce less resistance to air flow and provide an opened respiratory passageway.

Drugs for inhalation may be administered by a hand atomizer or a nebulizer. These devices break up the medication into a mist for more efficient inhalation.

The hand-held, metered-dose inhaler (MDI) is often used incorrectly, and the correct dose of medication is not delivered.

Nebulization may also result from the force of an oxygen stream or compressed air passed through the fluid in a nebulizer or an atomizer. This method is valuable for patients who require inhalation of a drug several times a day when the hand atomizer or nebulizer is fatiguing. The oxygen stream is also useful in the production of vapors when high humidity is needed continuously for long periods.

Documenting Medication Administration

The medication record is a legal document. Recording each dose of medication as soon as possible after it is given provides a documented record that can be consulted if there are any questions about whether the patient received the med-ication. The nurse should not record medications before they are given: if the medication is then not given, the medication record would falsely show that the patient received the medication. Different forms are used for recording medications. The name of the medication, dosage, route of administration, time given, and nurse's initials are noted on the form. The site used for an injection should be recorded. The nurse's full signature must appear on the form for initial identification. Other specific patient information may be required. For instance, the pulse rate may be recorded when administering some cardiac drugs, or a description of the effects on the patient's pain when administering analgesics may be recorded.

Omitted Drugs

Drugs may be omitted intentionally or inadvertently. The omission and the reason for it are documented on the patient's record. Drugs may be omitted intentionally for the following reasons:

- The patient is to have a diagnostic test and is to fast before the test. Oral drugs are usually omitted, or their administration is delayed, depending on the physician's orders.
- The problem for which the medication is intended no longer exists. For example, a laxative has been ordered for a patient. The patient has had a bowel movement and no longer needs the laxative. The laxative is then omitted.
- The patient is suspected of having an allergy to the medication. Any suspected allergy should be reported to the physician.

To reduce the incidence of medication errors, many healthcare facilities are using computerized medication administration record systems. These automated records give the pharmacy the capability to track statistical information, maintain inventory control of drugs, and integrate this information with the central billing system.

Refused Drugs

If the patient refuses a drug that is considered essential to the therapeutic regimen, the nurse should report this promptly. The nurse can often play an important role in determining the reason for the refusal and can help the patient accept needed drugs. If the patient is not persuaded by reasonable efforts and adamantly refuses a medication, it is unwise to continue urging the patient. Patients have the right to refuse therapy, and the nurse should recognize and respect that right. The refusal to take prescribed drugs and the manner in which the situation was managed should be described on the patient's record and reported according to agency policy.

Medication Errors

Nurses should take every precaution to avoid errors when administering therapeutic agents. Common types of medication errors include the following:

- Inappropriate prescribing of the drug (eg, incorrect dose, quantity, or route, or inadequate instruction)

Box 6
Guidelines for Nursing Care

Inserting Vaginal Suppository or Cream

- Fill a vaginal applicator with the prescribed amount of cream, or have a suppository ready.
- Lubricate the applicator with water, as necessary. A suppository may be lubricated with a water-soluble gel. Ordinarily, lubrication is unnecessary but may be used to reduce friction while inserting the applicator or suppository.
- Wear disposable gloves.
- Use clean aseptic technique to administer the medication.
- Spread the labia well with the fingers, and clean the area at the vaginal orifice with cotton balls and warm water to remove discharge, as necessary. With each cotton ball, use a single stroke moving from above the orifice downward toward the sacrum. These techniques prevent contamination of the vaginal orifice with debris surrounding the anus.
- Introduce the applicator gently in a rolling manner while directing it downward and backward to follow the normal contour of the vagina for its full length. Push the plunger to its full length, and then gently remove the applicator with the plunger depressed. After the applicator is properly positioned, the labia may be allowed to fall in place to free the nurse's hand for manipulating the plunger. Insert a suppository with gloved fingers well into the vagina.

- Ask the patient to remain in the supine position for 5 to 10 minutes after insertion.
- Offer the patient a perineal pad to collect excess drainage.
- Teach proper techniques to the patient who wants to administer vaginal suppositories and creams herself.

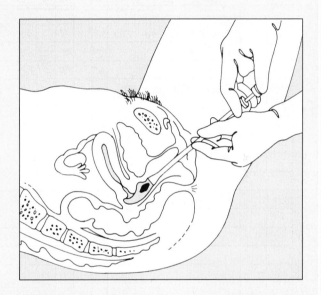

- Extra, omitted, or wrong doses
- Administration of a medication to a patient that was not ordered for him or her
- Administration of a drug by an incorrect route or rate
- Failure to give a medication within the prescribed time interval
- Incorrect preparation of a drug before giving it
- Improper technique when administering a drug
- Giving a drug that has deteriorated

Prompt acknowledgment of errors may minimize their possible detrimental effect. The immediate priority is the safety of the patient. The following steps are recommended when a medication error occurs:

1. Check the patient's condition immediately when the error is noted. Observe for the development of adverse effects related to the error.
2. Notify the nurse manager and the physician to discuss possible courses of action depending on the patient's condition.
3. Write a description of the error on the patient's medical record, including remedial steps that are taken.

4. Complete a special form for reporting errors, as dictated by agency policy. These forms, called *accident, incident,* or *unusual occurrence reports*, require an objective, complete account of the medication errors. Include the steps taken after the error was recognized. For legal reasons, it is essential that an error be described fully and accurately. Medication errors are a common allegation in nursing liability cases.

Although incident reports have a negative connotation for many nurses, they can provide vital information that can be used to prevent the error from being repeated in the future. The emphasis should be on the collaborative efforts necessary to provide safe patient care and decrease the incidence of errors. Peer review committees have proved effective in some healthcare settings.

Teaching About Medications and Abuse

Teaching about medications is an ongoing process and should begin as soon as the patient is admitted to the

CROZER-CHESTER MEDICAL CENTER
MEDICATION ADMINISTRATION + PARENTERAL THERAPY RECORD

FORM NS-MAR-1

Allergies:

Operative Date:
Procedure:

Penicillin

Legend for Injection Sites

RA - Right Arm   BT - Right Thigh
LA - Left Arm   LT - Left Thigh
RB - Right Buttock   R.Abd.- Right Abdomen
LB - Left Buttock   L.Abd.- Left Abdomen

STANDING ORDERS (MEDICATION ORDERED PER ROUTINE SCHEDULE OR WITH SPECIFIC NUMBER OF DOSES)

DATES, INJECTION SITES AND RN INITIALS

ORDER DATE & RN INIT.	EXP. DATE & TIME	MEDICATION, DOSAGE, FREQUENCY, ROUTE	HOURS	11/29 INJ. SITE	11/29 INIT.	11/30 INJ. SITE	11/30 INIT.	12/1 INJ. SITE	12/1 INIT.	12/2	12/3	12/4	12/5	12/6	12/7	12/8
11/29/01 SM		Digoxin 0.25 mg po QD	10 A	AC		AC		CL								
					AR ₌88		AR ₌92		AR ₌86							
11/29/01 SM		Lasix 20 mg QD po	10 A	AC		AC		CL								
11/29/01 SM		Trental 400 mg TIO Po	10 A	AC		AC		CL								
			2 P	AC		AC		CL								
			6 P	PR		PR		PR								
11/29/01 SM		Slow K+ po QD	10 A	AC		AC		(CL)								
11/29/01 SM		Serax 15 mg Po q. 8°	6 A	SP		SP		MS								
			2 P	AC		AC		CL								
			10 P	PR		PR		PR								
11/29/01 SM		Procardia 20 mg po TIO	10 A	AC		AC		CL								
			2 P	AC		AC		CL								
			6 P	PR		PR		PR								

SINGLE ORDERS (STAT, PRE-OP, ONE TIME DOSE, ON CALL, DIAGNOSTIC PREP)

ORDER DATE & RN INIT.	MEDICATION, DOSAGE, ROUTE	DATE	TIME	INJ. SITE	RN INIT.	ORDER DATE & RN INIT.	MEDICATION, DOSAGE, ROUTE	DATE	TIME	INJ. SITE	RN INIT.
11/29 PR	Dalmane 15 mg po now	11/29	11 P	–	PR						
11/30	Dulcolax Tab. ĩĩĩ po at 6 pm	11/30	6 P		PR						

Example of a medication record.

		PRN MEDICATIONS (ENTER DATE, TIME GIVEN, INJECTION SITE AND RN INITIALS)														
ORDER DATE & RN INIT.	EXP. DATE & TIME	MEDICATION, DOSES, FREQUENCY, ROUTE		DOSES GIVEN												
11/29/01 SM		Tylox tab ii po q 3° prn	DATE	11/29	11/30											
			TIME	1₉	3A											
			INJ. SITE													
			RN INIT.	AC	SP											
11/29/01 SM		Maalox 30cc po q 6° prn	DATE													
			TIME													
			INJ. SITE													
			RN INIT.													
			DATE													
			TIME													
			INJ. SITE													
			RN INIT.													

	PARENTERAL THERAPY			DOCUMENTATION FOR MEDICATION WITHHELD			
ORDER DATE & RN INIT.	I.V. SOLUTIONS	SCHEDULE	DATE	TIME	MEDICATION	REASON FOR WITHHOLDING	
11/29/01 SM	1000 cc D₅W	q. 8°	12/1	10A	Slow K tab ii	patient refused	
				RN IDENTIFICATION			
			INIT.	SIGNATURE	INIT.	SIGNATURE	INIT. SIGNATURE
			AC	a. Christopher RN			
			PR	P Rogers RN			
			SP	S. Pointer RN			
			CL	C. Lewis RN			

(Continued)

healthcare facility. In many cases, patients continue a prescribed medication regimen at home after discharge from the hospital. A factor that affects the patient's compliance to the medication regimen at home is education about the prescribed medications. Teaching should be tailored to the patient's level of understanding. Written instructions can be used as a reference for the patient and should include the following:

- The drug name and its intended effects
- Special instructions about taking the medication
- What to do when adverse effects occur
- Foods, beverages, and other medications that should be avoided while taking a medication
- Proper storage of the drug
- What to do if a dose is missed

Techniques of medication administration should be explained to the patient and family. Before discharge from a healthcare facility, the patient should practice the necessary techniques under the supervision of a nurse to acquire sufficient skill for safe administration. Many patients have learned to give themselves injections, as well as many other medications, when the teaching was planned well and the patient able and willing to learn.

The nurse should emphasize the importance of taking medications as prescribed and for as long as prescribed. A common error made by patients is simply omitting a drug, either through carelessness or because they believe that missing a dose is not important. Various aids are available to help nurses identify patients who are noncompliant and remind the patient to take his or her medication on schedule. Medication containers that beep when a dose is due to be taken, scratch-off dots on a medication label, and an electronic cap that signals dosage time and records each time the cap is removed are available as compliance aids. Patients should be advised to keep their medications with them when they travel. If luggage is lost or misplaced, refilling the prescription may be difficult.

The patient should be instructed not to alter the dosage without consulting the physician. Medications should not be discontinued when symptoms disappear. Drugs used to maintain health, such as those to control high blood pressure, need to be continued as ordered to avoid recurrence of symptoms.

Caution the patient not to share prescribed medications with other family members or with friends and neighbors. Inappropriate use of another person's drugs can have serious consequences.

Nurses have a teaching responsibility in relation to the abuse of any drug. Teaching may take place on an individual basis or on a family or community level. Drug abuse is a major public health concern worldwide, especially among teenagers and young adults. Not only is continued public and individual education indicated, but nurses are also expected to teach by setting high standards for their own behavior and the use of drugs. Because drug abuse is increasingly common and impairs healthcare providers, it is imperative that nurses observe, document, and intervene for the patient's safety, if drug abuse by a professional caregiver is suspected.

Bibliography

Abrams, A. (1998). *Clinical Drug Therapy* (5th ed.). Philadelphia: Lippincott Williams & Wilkins.

Beyea, S., & Nicoll, L. (1996). Back to basics: Administering IM injections the right way. *American Journal of Nursing, 96*(1), 34–35.

Chase, S. (1997). Pharmacology in practice: Back to basics. *RN, 60*(3), 24–26.

Covington, T., & Trattler, M. (1997). Bull's eye: Finding the right target for IM injections. *Nursing, 27*(1), 62–63.

DeBrew, J., Barba, B., & Tesh, A. (1998). Assessing medication knowledge and practices of older adults. *Home Healthcare Nurse, 16*(10), 686–691.

Edwards, J. (1997). Guarding against adverse drug events. *American Journal of Nursing, 97*(5), 26–31.

Eisenhauer, L., Nichols, L., Spencer, R., & Bergan, F. (1998). *Clinical Pharmacology and Nursing Management* (5th ed.). Philadelphia: Lippincott Williams & Wilkins.

Fleming, D. (1999). Challenging traditional insulin injection practices. *American Journal of Nursing, 99*(2), 72–74.

Gever, M. (1998). Transdermal patches: What's in a brand name? *Nursing, 28*(5), 58–59.

Guttadore, D. (1999). A quick way to identify compatible drugs. *RN, 62*(9), 53–55.

Kudzma, E. (1999). Culturally competent drug administration. *American Journal of Nursing, 99*(8), 46–51.

Howard, A., et al. (1997). Bevel-down superior to bevel-up in intradermal skin testing. *Annals of Allergy, Asthma, and Immunology, 78*(6), 594.

Kuhn, M. (1998). *Pharmacotherapeutics: A Nursing Process Approach* (4th ed.). Philadelphia: F. A. Davis.

Lazarou, J., Pomeranz, B., & Corey, P. (1998). Incidence of adverse drug reactions in hospitalized patients. *Journal of the American Medical Association, 279*, 1200–1205.

Lilley, L., & Guanci, R. (1996). Avoiding adverse reactions. *American Journal of Nursing, 96*(9), 18–19.

Lilley, L., & Guanci, R. (1997). Careful with the zeros! *American Journal of Nursing, 97*(5), 14.

McConnell, E. (1997). Using transdermal medication patches. *Nursing, 27*(7), 18.

McConnell, E. (1998a). Giving medications through an enteral feeding tube. *Nursing, 28*(3), 66.

McConnell, E. (1998b). Admixing drugs in a syringe. *Nursing, 28*(5), 20.

McConnell, E. (1998c). Applying transdermal ointments. *Nursing, 28*(10), 30.

McConnell, E. (1999). Administering a Z-track IM injection. *Nursing, 29*(1), 26.

McKenry, L., & Salerno, E. (1998). *Pharmacology in Nursing* (20th ed.). St. Louis: C. V. Mosby.

Miller, C. (1998). Frail elders: Handle with care when using medications. *Geriatric Nursing, 19*(4), 239–240.

Nagle, B. (1998). Low molecular weight heparin. *RN, 61*(4), 40–43.

North American Nursing Diagnosis Association. (1999). *Nursing diagnoses: Definitions and classification 1999–2000,* Philadelphia: Author.

Pavlovich-Danis, S. (1999). Ethnicity and culture vary medicinal effects. *Nursing Spectrum, 8*(20), 18–19.

Richards, J., & Creamer, L. (1999). Med errors: Solving the microgram/kilogram puzzle. *American Journal of Nursing, 99*(10), 12.

Segbefia, I., & Mallet, L. (1997). Are your patients taking their medications correctly? *Nursing, 27*(4), 58–60.

Shirrell, D., Gibbar-Clements, T., Dooley, R., & Free, C. (1999). Understanding therapeutic drug monitoring. *American Journal of Nursing, 99*(1), 42–44.

Shuster, J. (1997). Looking out for adverse drug reactions. *Nursing, 27*(11), 34–39.

Skolnick, A. (1997). FDA sets geriatric drug use labeling deadlines. *Journal of the American Medical Association, 278*(16), 1302.

Wendt, D. (1998). Evaluation of medication management interventions for the elderly. *Home Healthcare Nurse, 16*(9), 612–617.

PROCEDURE 1

Removing Medication From an Ampule

Equipment

Sterile syringe and needle (size depends on medication being administered and patient)

Ampule of medication
Medication Kardex or computer-generated MAR

Alcohol swab or gauze pad
Filter needle (optional)

Action	Rationale
1. Gather equipment. Check the medication order against the original physician's order according to agency policy.	This comparison helps to identify errors that may have occurred when orders were transcribed.
2. Wash your hands.	Handwashing deters the spread of microorganisms.
3. Tap the stem of the ampule or twist your wrist quickly while holding the ampule vertically.	This facilitates movement of medication in the stem to the body of the ampule.
4. Wrap a small gauze pad or dry alcohol swab around the neck of the ampule.	This protects the nurse's fingers from the glass as the ampule is broken.
5. Use a snapping motion to break off the top of the ampule along the prescored line at its neck. Always break away from your body.	This protects the nurse's face and fingers from any shattered glass fragments.

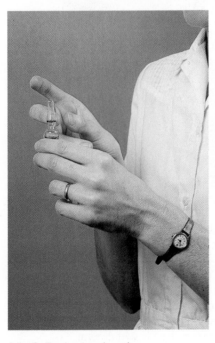

Action 3: Tapping stem of ampule.

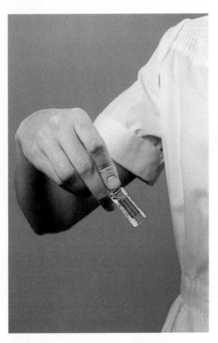

Action 3: Twisting motion of wrist while holding ampule.

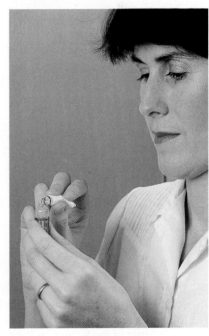

Action 5: Snapping off top of ampule.

6. Remove the cap from the needle by pulling it straight off. Insert the needle into the ampule, being careful not to touch the rim. (Some agencies recommend use of a filter needle when withdrawing solution from an ampule.)	The rim of the ampule is considered contaminated. (Use of a filter needle prevents the accidental withdrawing of small glass particles with the medication.)

(continued)

PROCEDURE 1

Removing Medication From an Ampule (Continued)

7. Withdraw medication in the amount ordered. Do not inject air into solutions. Use either of the following methods:

   a. Insert the tip of the needle into the ampule, which is *upright* on a flat surface, and withdraw fluid into the syringe. Touch plunger at knob only.

   b. Insert the tip of the needle into the ampule and *invert* the ampule. Keep the needle centered and not touching the sides of the ampule. Remove the prescribed amount of medication. Touch plunger at knob only.

The contents of the ampule are not under pressure; therefore, air is unnecessary and will cause the contents to overflow. Handling plunger at knob only will keep shaft of plunger sterile.

Surface tension holds the fluid in the ampule when inverted. If the needle touches the sides or is removed and then reinserted into the ampule, surface tension is broken, and fluid runs out. Handling plunger at knob only will keep shaft of plunger sterile.

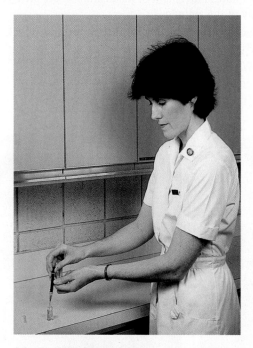

Action 7a: Withdrawing medication from upright ampule.

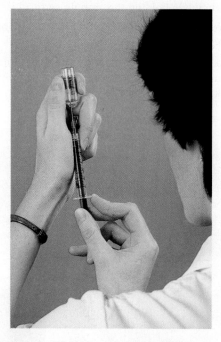

Action 7b: Withdrawing medication from inverted ampule. (PHOTOS © KEN KASPER.)

8. Do not expel any air bubbles that may form in the solution. Wait until the needle has been withdrawn to tap the syringe and expel the air carefully. Check the amount of medication in the syringe and discard any surplus.

9. Discard the ampule in a suitable container after comparing with the medication Kardex.

10. Replace the cap carefully over the needle on the syringe.

11. Wash your hands.

Ejecting air into the solution increases pressure in the ampule and can force the medication to spill out over the ampule. Ampules may have overfill. Careful measurement ensures that correct dose is withdrawn.

If all of the medication has been removed from the ampule, it must be discarded because there is no way to maintain sterility of contents in an unopened ampule.

This prevents contamination of the needle and protects the nurse against inadvertent needlesticks. A one-handed recap method may be used.

Handwashing deters the spread of microorganisms.

PROCEDURE 2

Removing Medication From a Vial

Equipment

Sterile syringe and needle (size depends on medication being administered and patient)

Vial of medication
Medication Kardex or computer-generated MAR

Alcohol swab
Filter needle (optional)

Action	Rationale
1. Gather equipment. Check medication order against the original physician's order according to agency policy.	This comparison helps to identify errors that may have occurred when orders were transcribed.
2. Wash your hands.	Handwashing deters the spread of microorganisms.
3. Remove the metal or plastic cap on the vial that protects the rubber stopper.	The metal or plastic cap prevents contamination of the rubber top.
4. Swab the rubber top with the alcohol swab.	Alcohol removes surface bacteria contamination. This is not necessary the first time the rubber stopper is entered, but subsequent reentries into the vial require the use of alcohol cleansing.
5. Remove the cap from the needle by pulling it straight off. (Some agencies recommend use of a filter needle when withdrawing premixed medication from multi-dose vials.) Draw back an amount of air into the syringe that is equal to the specific dose of medication to be withdrawn.	Before fluid is removed, injection of an equal amount of air is required to prevent the formation of a partial vacuum because a vial is a sealed container. If not enough air is injected, the negative pressure makes it difficult to withdraw the medication. (Use of a filter needle prevents any solid material from being withdrawn through the needle.)
6. Pierce the rubber stopper in the center with the needle tip and inject the measured air into the space above the solution. (Do not inject air into the solution.) The vial may be positioned upright on a flat surface or inverted.	Air bubbled through the solution could result in withdrawal of an inaccurate amount of medication.

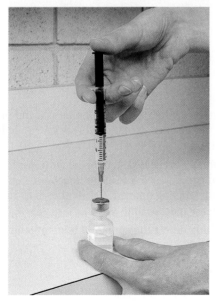

Action 6: Injecting air with vial upright.

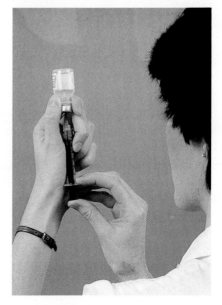

Action 6: Injecting air with vial inverted and needle above solution.

(continued)

PROCEDURE 2

Removing Medication From a Vial (Continued)

7. Invert the vial and withdraw the needle tip slightly so that it is below the fluid level.

8. Draw up the prescribed amount of medication while holding the syringe at eye level and vertically. Be careful to touch the plunger at knob only.

9. If any air bubbles accumulate in the syringe, tap the barrel of the syringe sharply and move the needle past the fluid into the air space to reinject the air bubble into the vial. Return the needle tip to the solution and continue withdrawal of the medication.

This prevents air from being aspirated into the syringe.

Holding the syringe at eye level facilitates accurate reading, and the vertical position makes removal of air bubbles from the syringe easy. Handling plunger at knob only will keep shaft of plunger sterile.

Removal of air bubbles is necessary to ensure accurate dose of medication.

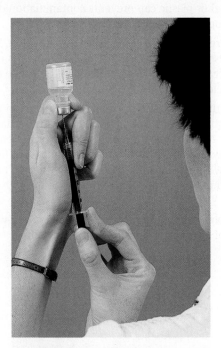

Action 8: Withdrawing medication at eye level.

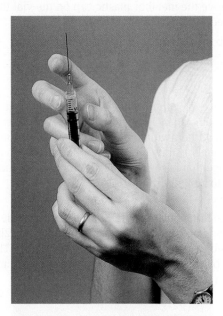

Action 9: Tapping to remove air bubbles. (PHOTOS © KEN KASPER.)

10. After the correct dose is withdrawn, remove the needle from the vial and carefully replace the cap over the needle.

11. If a multidose vial is being used, store the vial containing the remaining medication according to agency policy.

12. Wash your hands.

This prevents contamination of the needle and protects the nurse against accidental needlesticks. A one-handed recap method may be used.

Because the vial is sealed, the medication inside remains sterile and can be used for future injections. Some agencies require labeling opened vials with a date and limiting its use after a specific time period.

Handwashing deters the spread of microorganisms.

PROCEDURE 3

Mixing Insulins in One Syringe

Equipment

Two vials of insulin
Medication Kardex or computer-
     generated MAR

Sterile insulin syringe with 25-gauge
     or 27-gauge needle
Alcohol swabs

Action	Rationale
1. Gather equipment. Check medication order against the original physician's order according to agency policy.	This comparison helps to identify errors that may have occurred when orders were transcribed.
2. Wash your hands.	Handwashing deters the spread of microorganisms.
3. If necessary, remove the metal cap that protects the rubber stopper on each vial.	The metal cap prevents contamination of the rubber top.
4. If insulin is a suspension (NPH, Lente), shake the vial vigorously.	Rolling a vial does not adequately mix NPH or LENTE insulin and may result in an inconsistent dose. Regular insulin or clear insulin does not need to be mixed before withdrawal.
5. Cleanse the rubber tops with alcohol swabs.	It is questionable whether cleaning with alcohol actually disinfects or, instead, transfers resident bacteria from the hands to another surface. Because it is difficult in a healthcare facility to keep an insulin vial in its original box as recommended, cleansing with alcohol will most likely continue.
6. Remove cap from needle. Inject air into the modified insulin preparation (eg, NPH insulin). Touch plunger at knob only. Use an amount of air equal to the amount of medication to be withdrawn. Do not allow the needle to touch the medication in the vial. Remove the needle.	Regular, or short-acting, insulin should never be contaminated with NPH or any insulin modified with added protein. Placing air in the NPH insulin first without allowing the needle to contact the insulin ensures that regular insulin is not contaminated with the additional protein in the NPH. Handling the plunger by the knob only assures sterility of shaft of plunger.
7. Inject air into the clear insulin without additional protein (eg, regular insulin). Use an amount of air equal to the amount of medication to be withdrawn.	An equal amount of air must be injected into the vacuum to allow easy withdrawal of medication.

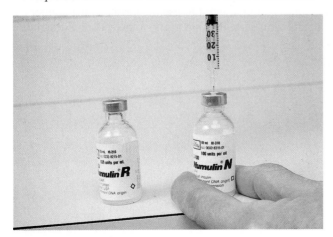

Action 6: Injecting air into modified insulin preparation.

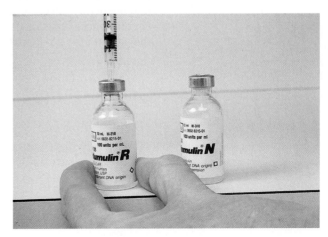

Action 7: Injecting air into clear insulin.

(*continued*)

PROCEDURE 3

Mixing Insulins in One Syringe (Continued)

8. Invert the vial of clear insulin and aspirate the amount prescribed. Remove the needle from the vial.

Regular insulin that contains no additional protein is not contaminated by insulin that contains globulin or protamine.

9. Cleanse the rubber top of the modified insulin vial. Insert the needle into this vial, invert it, and withdraw the medication. Carefully replace the cap over the needle.

Previous addition of air eliminates need to create positive pressure. Capping the needle prevents contamination and protects the nurse against accidental needlesticks. A one-handed recap method may be used.

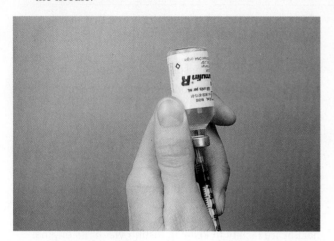

Action 8: Withdrawing clear insulin.

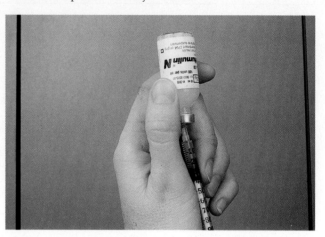

Action 9: Withdrawing modified insulin. (PHOTOS © KEN KASPER.)

10. Store the vials according to agency recommendations.

Insulin need not be refrigerated but must be protected from temperature extremes.

11. Wash your hands.

Handwashing deters the spread of microorganisms.

Special Considerations

An insulin-dependent diabetic patient who is visually impaired may find it helpful to use a magnifying apparatus that fits around the syringe.

An insulin-cartridge pen (the Novalin Pen) is available that allows the patient to dial the correct dose of insulin and press a button to release the dose quickly through a short, fine, 27-gauge needle.

Before attempting to explain or demonstrate devices that aid low-vision diabetic patients to prepare their medication, the nurse should attempt to use the device under similar circumstances. Practice using the aid with a blindfold in place, to detect any difficulties the patient may experience.

PROCEDURE 4

Administering Oral Medications

Equipment

Medication Kardex or computer-generated MAR	Medication cart or tray Medication cups (disposable)	Straws Water or juice

Action	**Rationale**
1. Gather equipment. Check each medication order against the original physician's order according to agency policy. Clarify any inconsistencies. Check the patient's chart for allergies.	This comparison helps to identify errors that may have occurred when orders were transcribed. The physician's order is the legal record of medication orders for each agency.
2. Know the actions, special nursing considerations, safe-dose ranges, purpose of administration, and adverse effects of medications to be administered.	This knowledge aids the nurse in evaluating the therapeutic effect of the medication in relation to the patient's disorder and can also be used to educate the patient about their medications.
3. Wash your hands.	Handwashing prevents the spread of microorganisms.
4. Move the medication cart to the outside of the patient's room or prepare for administration in the medication area.	Organization facilitates error-free administration and saves time.
5. Unlock the medication cart or drawer.	Locking of the cart or drawer safeguards each patient's medication supply.
6. Prepare medications for one patient at a time.	This prevents errors in medication administration.
7. Select the proper medication from the drawer or stock and compare with the Kardex or order. Check expiration dates and perform calculations if necessary.	Comparison of medication to physician's order reduces errors in medication administration. Verify calculations with another nurse if necessary. This is the *first* safety check.
a. Place unit dose–packaged medications in a disposable cup. *Do not open wrapper* until at bedside. Keep narcotics and medications that require special nursing assessments in a separate container.	The label is needed for an additional safety check. Prerequisites to giving certain medications may include monitoring of certain vital signs.
b. When removing tablets or capsules from a bottle, pour the necessary number into the bottle cap and then place the tablets in a medication cup. Break only scored tablets, if necessary, to obtain the proper dose.	Pouring medication into the cap allows for easy return of excess medication to bottle. Pouring tablets or capsules into the nurse's hand is unsanitary.
c. Hold liquid medication bottles with the label against the palm. Use the appropriate measuring device when pouring liquids, and read the amount of medication at the bottom of the meniscus at eye level. Wipe the lip of the bottle with a paper towel.	Accuracy is possible when the appropriate measuring device is used and then read accurately. Liquid that may drip onto the label makes the label difficult to read.
8. Recheck each medication package or preparation with the order as it is poured.	This is a *second* check to guard against a medication error.
9. When all medications for one client have been prepared, recheck once again with the medication order before taking them to the client.	This is a *third* check to ensure accuracy and to prevent errors.

(continued)

PROCEDURE 4

Administering Oral Medications (Continued)

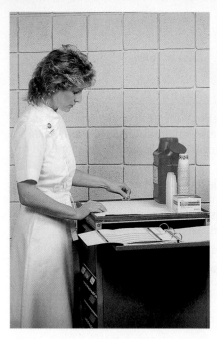

Action 5: Unlocking medication cart.

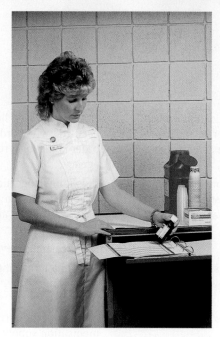

Action 7: Comparing medication with Kardex or order.

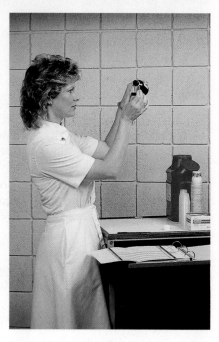

Action 7c: Measuring at eye level.

10. Transport medications to the patient's bedside carefully, and keep the medications in sight at all times.

Careful handling and close observation prevent accidental or deliberate disarrangement of medications.

11. See that the patient receives medications at the correct time.

Check agency policy, which may allow for administration within a period of 30 minutes before or 30 minutes after designated time.

12. Identify the patient carefully. There are three correct ways to do this:
    a. Check the name on the patient's identification band.
    b. Ask the patient his or her name.

    c. Verify the patient's identification with a staff member who knows the patient.

Identifying the patient is the nurse's responsibility to guard against error.
This is the most reliable method. Replace the identification band if it is missing or inaccurate in any way.
This requires a response from the patient, but illness and strange surroundings often cause patients to be confused.
This is another way to double check identity. Do not use the name on the door or over the bed because these may be inaccurate.

13. Complete necessary assessments before administration of medications. Check allergy bracelet or ask patient about allergies. Explain the purpose and action of each medication to the patient.

Assessment is a prerequisite to administration of medications.

14. Assist the patient to an upright or lateral position.

Swallowing is facilitated by proper positioning. An upright or side-lying position protects the patient from aspiration.

PROCEDURE 4

Administering Oral Medications (Continued)

15. Administer medications:
    a. Offer water or other permitted fluids with pills, capsules, tablets, and some liquid medications.

    b. Ask the patient's preference regarding medications to be taken by hand or in a cup and one at a time or all at once.
    c. If the capsule or tablet falls to the floor, it must be discarded and a new one administered.
    d. Record any fluid intake if intake and output measurement is ordered.
16. Remain with the patient until each medication is swallowed. Unless the nurse has seen the patient swallow the drug, it cannot be recorded that the drug was administered.

Liquids facilitate swallowing of solid drugs. Some liquid drugs are intended to adhere to the pharyngeal area, in which case liquid is not offered with the medication. This encourages the patient's participation in taking the medications.

This prevents contamination.

This provides for accurate documentation.

The patient's chart is a legal record. Only with a physician's order can medications be left at the bedside.

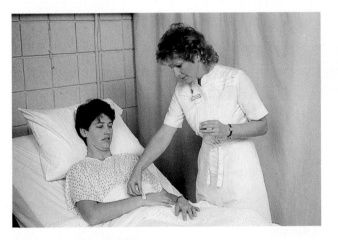

Action 12a: Checking patient identity.

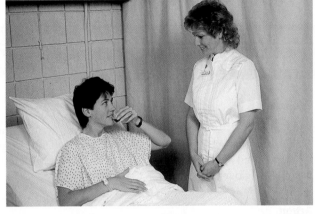

Action 16: Observing patient swallowing medication. (PHOTOS © KEN KASPER.)

17. Wash your hands.
18. Record each medication given on the medication chart or record using the required format.
    a. If the drug was refused or omitted, record this in the appropriate area on the medication record.
    b. Recording of administration of a narcotic requires additional documentation on a narcotic record stating drug count and other specific information.
19. Check on the patient within 30 minutes to verify response to medication.

Handwashing prevents the spread of microorganisms.

Prompt recording avoids the possibility of accidentally repeating the administration of the drug.
This verifies the reason medication was omitted.

Controlled substance laws necessitate careful recording of narcotic use.

This provides opportunity for further documentation and additional assessment of effectiveness of pain relief and adverse effects of medications.

Age Considerations

Special devices are available in a pharmacy to ensure accurate dose calculations for young children and infants.

Elderly patients with arthritis may have difficulty opening childproof caps. On request, the pharmacist can substitute a cap that is easier to open. A rubber band twisted around the cap may provide a more secure grip for older patients.

(continued)

PROCEDURE 4

Administering Oral Medications (Continued)

The FDA has received reports of infants choking on the plastic caps that fit on the end of syringes used to administer oral medication. They recommend: removal and disposal of caps before giving syringes to patients or families, caution family caregivers to dispose of caps on syringes they buy over the counter, and report any problems with syringe caps to the FDA.

Home Care Considerations

Encourage the patient to discard outdated prescription medications.

Discuss safe storage of medications when there are children and pets in the environment.

Special Considerations

If the patient questions a medication order or states the medication is different from the usual dose, *always* recheck and clarify with the original order before giving medication.

If the patient's level of consciousness is altered or his or her swallowing is impaired, check with the physician to clarify the route of administration or alternative forms of medication.

Patients with poor vision can request labels printed with larger type on medication containers. A magnifying lens also may prove helpful.

PROCEDURE 5

Administering an Intradermal Injection

Equipment

Medication
Medication Kardex or computer-
  generated MAR
Disposable gloves

Sterile syringe and needle (size
  depends on medication being
  administered and patient)

Alcohol swab
Acetone and 2 × 2 sterile gauze
  square (optional)

Action	Rationale
1. Assemble equipment and check the physician's order.	This ensures that the patient receives the right medication at the right time by the proper route. Many intradermal drugs are potent allergens and may cause a significant reaction if given in an incorrect dose.
2. Explain the procedure to the patient.	Explanation encourages cooperation and reduces apprehension.
3. Wash your hands. Don disposable gloves.	Handwashing deters the spread of microorganisms. Gloves act as a barrier and protect the nurse's hands from accidental exposure to blood during the injection procedure.
4. If necessary, withdraw medication from an ampule or vial as described in Procedures 1 and 2.	
5. Select an area on the inner aspect of the forearm that is not heavily pigmented or covered with hair. The upper chest or upper back beneath the scapulae also are sites for intradermal injections.	The forearm is a convenient and easy location for introducing an agent intradermally. Hair or lesions at the injection site may interfere with assessments of skin changes at the site.
6. Cleanse the area with an alcohol swab while wiping with a firm, circular motion and moving outward from the injection site. Allow the skin to dry. If the skin is oily, clean the area with a pledget moistened with acetone.	Pathogens on the skin can be forced into the tissues by the needle. Introducing alcohol into tissues irritates the tissues and is uncomfortable for the patient. Acetone is effective for removing oily substances from the skin.

PROCEDURE 5

Administering an Intradermal Injection (Continued)

7. Use the nondominant hand to spread the skin taut over the injection site.

Taut skin provides an easy entrance into intradermal tissue.

8. Remove the needle cap with the nondominant hand by pulling it straight off.

The cap protects the needle from contact with micro-organisms. This technique lessens the risk of an accidental needlestick.

9. Place the needle almost flat against the patient's skin, bevel side up, and insert the needle into the skin so that the point of the needle can be seen through the skin. Insert the needle only about ⅛ inch.

Intradermal tissue is entered when the needle is held as nearly parallel to the skin as possible and is inserted about ⅛ inch.

10. Slowly inject the agent while watching for a small wheal or blister to appear. If none appears, withdraw the needle slightly.

If a small wheal or blister appears, the agent is in intradermal tissue.

11. Withdraw the needle quickly at the same angle that it was inserted.

Withdrawing the needle quickly and at the angle at which it entered the skin minimizes tissue damage and discomfort for the patient.

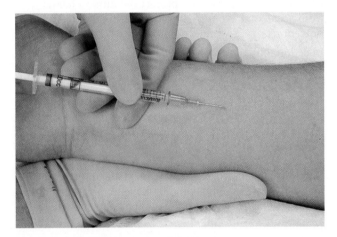

Action 9: Inserting the needle almost level with the skin.

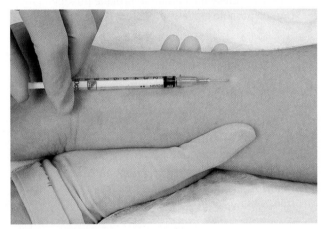

Action 10: Observing for wheal while injecting medication.

12. Do not massage the area after removing the needle.

Massaging the area where an intradermal injection is given may interfere with test results by spreading medication to underlying subcutaneous tissue.

13. Do not recap the used needle. Discard the needle and syringe in the appropriate receptacle.

Proper disposal of the needle protects the nurse from accidental injection. Most accidental puncture wounds occur when recapping needles.

14. Assist the patient to a position of comfort.

This provides for the well-being of the patient.

15. Remove gloves and dispose of them properly. Wash your hands.

Handwashing deters the spread of microorganisms.

16. Chart the administration of the medication.

Accurate documentation is necessary to prevent medication error.

17. Observe the area for signs of a reaction at ordered intervals, usually at 24- to 72-hour periods. Inform the patient of this inspection. In some agencies, a circle may be drawn on the skin around the injection site.

This easily identifies the site of the intradermal injection and allows for careful observation of the exact area.

Special Considerations   Recent research has indicated that a bevel-down technique may be preferable when performing skin testing (Howard et al., 1997).

PROCEDURE 6

Administering a Subcutaneous Injection

Equipment

Medication
Medication Kardex or computer-
generated MAR

A sterile syringe and needle (size
depends on medication being
administered and patient)

Alcohol swabs
Disposable gloves

Action	Rationale
1. Assemble equipment and check the physician's order.	This ensures that the patient receives the right medication at the right time by the proper route.
2. Explain the procedure to the patient.	An explanation encourages patient cooperation and reduces apprehension.
3. Wash your hands.	Handwashing deters the spread of microorganisms.
4. If necessary, withdraw medication from an ampule or vial as described in Procedures 1 and 2.	
5. Identify the patient carefully. See Procedure 4, action 12. Close the curtain to provide privacy. Don disposable gloves.	It is the nurse's responsibility to guard against error. Gloves act as a barrier and protect the nurse's hands from accidental exposure to blood during the injection procedure.

6. Have the patient assume a position appropriate for the most commonly used sites:
  a. Outer aspect of upper arm—the patient's arm should be relaxed and at the side of the body.
  b. Anterior thighs—the patient may sit or lie with the leg relaxed.
  c. Abdomen—the patient may lie in a semi-recumbent position.
	Injection into a tense muscle causes discomfort.

7. Locate the site of choice according to directions given in this Atlas. Ensure that the area is not tender and is free of lumps or nodules.	Good visualization is necessary to establish the correct location of the site and avoid damage to tissues. Nodules or lumps may indicate a previous injection site where absorption was inadequate.
8. Clean the area around the injection site with an alcohol swab. Use a firm, circular motion while moving outward from the injection site. Allow the antiseptic to dry. Leave the alcohol swab in a clean area for reuse when withdrawing the needle.	Friction helps to clean the skin. A clean area is contaminated when a soiled object is rubbed over its surface.
9. Remove the needle cap with the nondominant hand, pulling it straight off.	The cap protects the needle from contact with microorganisms. This technique lessens the risk of an accidental needlestick.
10. Grasp and bunch the area surrounding the injection site or spread the skin at the site.	This provides for easy, less painful entry into the subcutaneous tissue. The decision to pinch or spread tissue at the injection site depends on the size of the patient. If the patient is thin, skin needs to be bunched to create a skinfold.
11. Hold the syringe in the dominant hand between the thumb and forefinger. Inject the needle quickly at an angle at 45 to 90 degrees, depending on the amount and turgor of the tissue and the length of the needle, as shown.	Subcutaneous tissue is abundant in well-nourished, well-hydrated people and spare in emaciated, dehydrated, or very thin persons. For a thin person, it is best to insert the needle at a 45-degree angle.

Administering a Subcutaneous Injection (Continued)

12. After the needle is in place, release the tissue and immediately move your nondominant hand to steady the lower end of the syringe. Slide your dominant hand to the tip of the barrel.

Injecting the solution into compressed tissues results in pressure against nerve fibers and creates discomfort. The nondominant hand secures the syringe and allows for smooth aspiration.

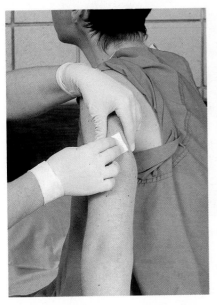

Action 8: Cleaning injection site.

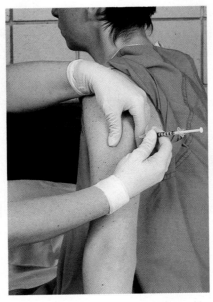

Action 10: Bunching tissue around injection site.

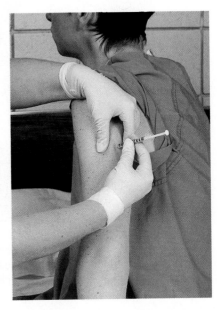

Action 11: Inserting needle.

13. Aspirate, if recommended, by pulling back gently on the plunger of the syringe to determine whether the needle is in a blood vessel. If blood appears, the needle should be withdrawn, the medication syringe and needle discarded, and a new syringe with new medication prepared. *Do not aspirate when giving insulin or heparin.*

14. If no blood appears, inject the solution slowly.

15. Withdraw the needle quickly at the same angle at which it was inserted, as shown.

16. Massage the area gently with the alcohol swab. (Do not massage a subcutaneous heparin or insulin injection site.)

Discomfort and possibly a serious reaction may occur if a drug intended for subcutaneous use is injected into a vein. Heparin is an anticoagulant and may cause bruising if aspirated. Because the insulin needle is so small, aspiration after insulin has proved unreliable in predicting needle placement.

Rapid injection of the solution creates pressure in the tissues, resulting in discomfort.

Slow withdrawal of the needle pulls the tissues and causes discomfort. Applying countertraction around the injection site helps to prevent pulling on the tissue as the needle is withdrawn. Removing the needle at the same angle at which it was inserted minimizes tissue damage and discomfort for the patient.

Massaging helps to distribute the solution and hastens its absorption. Massaging the site of a heparin injection causes additional bruising. Massaging after an insulin injection may contribute to unpredictable absorption of the medication.

(continued)

Administering a Subcutaneous Injection (Continued)

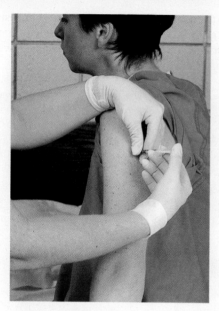

Action 14: Injecting medication.

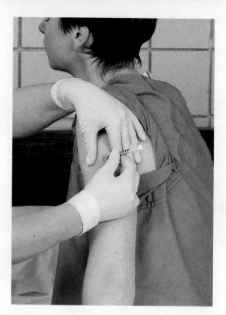

Action 15: Withdrawing needle. (PHOTOS © B. PROUD.)

17. Do not recap the used needle. Discard the needle and syringe in the appropriate receptacle.

Proper disposal of the needle protects the nurse from accidental injection. Most accidental puncture wounds occur when recapping needles.

18. Assist the patient to a position of comfort.

This provides for the well-being of the patient.

19. Remove gloves and dispose of them properly. Wash your hands.

Handwashing deters the spread of microorganisms.

20. Chart the administration of the medication.

Accurate documentation is necessary to prevent medication error.

21. Evaluate the response of the patient to medication within an appropriate time frame.

Reaction to medication given by the parenteral route may occur within 15 to 30 minutes after injection.

Home Care Considerations   According to the American Diabetes Association, reuse of insulin syringes in this setting appears safe. Once the needle is dull, it should be discarded (usually after 2 to 10 uses). Only in this situation and setting, can the needle be recapped between uses (Fleming, 1999).

PROCEDURE 7

Administering an Intramuscular Injection

Equipment

Medication
Medication Kardex or computer-
generated MAR

Sterile syringe and needle (size
depends on medication being
administered and patient)

Alcohol swab
Dry sponge
Disposable gloves

Action	Rationale
1. Assemble equipment and check the physician's order.	This ensures that the patient receives the right medication at the right time by the proper route.
2. Explain the procedure to the patient.	Explanation encourages cooperation and alleviates apprehension.
3. Wash your hands.	Handwashing deters the spread of microorganisms.
4. If necessary, withdraw medication from an ampule or vial as described in Procedures 1 and 2.	
5. Do not add air to the syringe.	The addition of air to the syringe is potentially dangerous and may result in an overdose of medication.

6. Provide for privacy. Have the patient assume a position appropriate for the site selected.
  a. Ventrogluteal—the patient may lie on the back or side with the hip and knee flexed.
  b. Vastus lateralis—the patient may lie on the back or may assume a sitting position.
  c. Deltoid—the patient may sit or lie with arm relaxed.
  d. Dorsogluteal—the patient may lie prone with toes pointing inward or on the side with the upper leg flexed and placed in front of the lower leg.
	Injection into a tense muscle causes discomfort.

7. Locate the site of choice according to directions given in this chapter and ensure that the area is nontender and free of lumps or nodules. Don disposable gloves.	Good visualization is necessary to establish the correct location of the site and avoid damage to tissues. Nodules or lumps may indicate a previous injection site where absorption was inadequate. Gloves act as a barrier and protect the nurse's hands from accidental exposure to blood during the injection procedure.
8. Clean the area thoroughly with an alcohol swab, using friction. Allow alcohol to dry.	Pathogens present on the skin and alcohol can be forced into the tissues by the needle.
9. Remove the needle cap by pulling it straight off.	The cap protects the needle from contact with microorganisms. This technique lessens the risk of an accidental needlestick and also prevents inadvertently unscrewing the needle from the barrel of the syringe.
10. Displace the skin in a Z-track manner or spread the skin at the site using your nondominant hand.	This makes the tissue taut and minimizes discomfort. Z-track prevents seepage of the medication into the needle track and is less painful.
11. Hold the syringe in your dominant hand between the thumb and forefinger. Quickly dart the needle into the tissue at a 90-degree angle.	A quick injection is less painful. Inserting the needle at a 90-degree angle facilitates entry into muscle tissue.

(continued)

Administering an Intramuscular Injection (Continued)

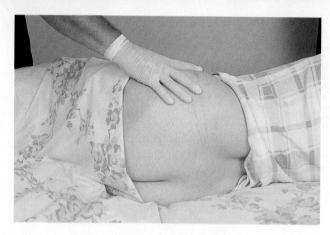

Action 7: Identifying landmarks for ventrogluteal injection site.

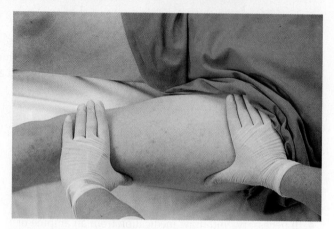

Action 7: Identifying vastus lateralis injection site.

12. As soon as the needle is in place, use your nondominant hand to hold the lower end of the syringe. Slide your dominant hand to the tip of the barrel.

13. Aspirate by slowly (for at least 5 seconds) pulling back on the plunger to determine whether the needle is in a blood vessel. If blood is aspirated, discard the needle, syringe, and medication, prepare a new sterile setup, and inject another site.

14. If no blood is aspirated, inject the solution slowly (10 seconds per mL of medication).

This acts to steady the syringe and allows for smooth aspiration.

Discomfort and possibly a serious reaction may occur if a drug intended for intramuscular use is injected into a vein. Allowing slow aspiration facilitates back-flow of blood even if needle is in a small, low-flow blood vessel.

Injecting slowly helps to reduce discomfort by allowing time for the solution to disperse in the tissues.

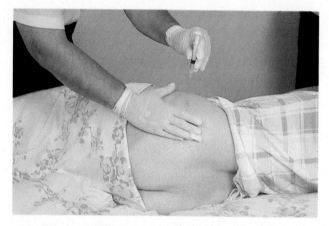

Actions 10 and 11: Displacing tissue in a Z-track manner and darting needle into tissue.

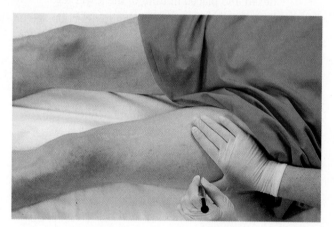

Actions 10 and 11: Spreading the skin at vastus lateralis site and darting needle into the tissue. (PHOTOS © B. PROUD.)

PROCEDURE 7

Administering an Intramuscular Injection (Continued)

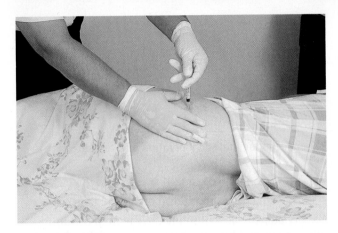

Action 13: Aspirating.

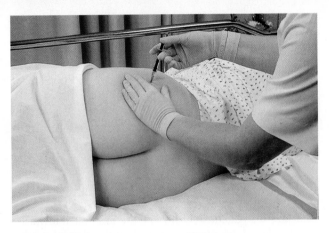

Action 14: Injecting.

15. Remove the needle slowly and steadily. Release displaced tissue if Z-track technique was used.

Slow withdrawal allows the medication to begin to be diffused through the muscle.

16. Apply gentle pressure at the site with a small, dry sponge.

Light pressure causes less trauma and irritation to the tissues.

17. Do not recap the used needle. Discard the needle and syringe in the appropriate receptacle.

Proper disposal of the needle protects the nurse from accidental injection. Most accidental puncture wounds occur when recapping needles.

18. Assist the patient to a position of comfort. Encourage patient to exercise leg if possible.

Exercise promotes absorption of the medication.

19. Remove gloves and dispose of them properly. Wash your hands.

Handwashing deters the spread of microorganisms.

20. Chart the administration of the medication.

Accurate documentation is necessary to prevent medication error.

21. Evaluate the response of the patient to the medication within an appropriate time frame. Assess site, if possible, within 2–4 hours after administration.

Reaction to medication given by the parenteral route is a possibility. Assessment also allows for visualization of the site for any untoward effects.

Age Considerations   Safe administration of an intramuscular injection into an infant's vastus lateralis muscle may require use of a 1-inch needle rather than the commonly used ⅝-inch needle. A 1-inch needle consistently allows penetration into the muscle and safe administration of the medication.

PROCEDURE 8

Administering an Eye Irrigation

Equipment

Sterile irrigating solution (warmed to 37°C [98.6°F])

Sterile irrigation set (sterile container and irrigating or bulb syringe)

Cotton balls

Emesis basin or irrigation basin

Disposable gloves

Waterproof pad

Towel

Action	Rationale
1. Explain procedure to patient.	Explanation facilitates cooperation and reassures the patient.
2. Assemble equipment.	This provides for an organized approach to the task.
3. Wash your hands.	Handwashing deters the spread of microorganisms.
4. Have the patient sit or lie with the head tilted toward the side of the affected eye. Protect the patient and the bed with a waterproof pad.	Gravity aids the flow of solution away from the unaffected eye and from the inner canthus of the affected eye toward the outer canthus.
5. Don disposable gloves. Clean the lids and the lashes with a cotton ball moistened with normal saline or the solution ordered for the irrigation. Wipe from the inner to the outer canthus. Discard the cotton ball after each wipe.	Materials lodged on the lids or in the lashes may be washed into the eye. This cleaning motion protects the nasolacrimal duct and the other eye.
6. Place the curved basin at the cheek on the side of the affected eye to receive the irrigating solution. If the patient is sitting up, ask him or her to support the basin.	Gravity aids the flow of solution.
7. Expose the lower conjunctival sac and hold the upper lid open with your nondominant hand.	The solution is directed onto the lower conjunctival sac because the cornea is sensitive and easily injured. This also prevents reflex blinking.

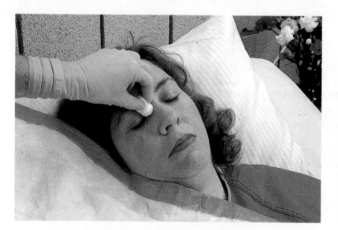

Action 5: Cleaning lids and lashes from inside of eye to outside.

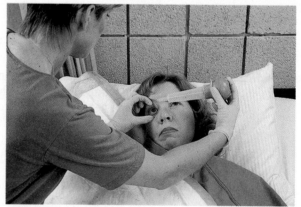

Action 7: Preparing to irrigate the eye. (PHOTOS © B. PROUD.)

8. Hold the irrigator about 2.5 cm (1 inch) from the eye. Direct the flow of the solution from the inner to the outer canthus along the conjunctival sac.

This minimizes the risk for injury to the cornea. Solution directed toward the outer canthus helps to prevent the spread of contamination from the eye to the lacrimal sac, the lacrimal duct, and the nose.

PROCEDURE 8

Administering an Eye Irrigation (Continued)

Action	Rationale
9. Irrigate until the solution is clear or all of the solution has been used. Use only sufficient force to remove secretions gently from the conjunctiva. Avoid touching any part of the eye with the irrigating tip.	Directing solutions with force may cause injury to the tissues of the eye as well as to the conjunctiva. Touching the eye is uncomfortable for the patient.
10. Have the patient close the eye periodically during the procedure.	Movement of the eye when the lids are closed helps to move secretions from the upper to the lower conjunctival sac.
11. Dry the area after the irrigation with cotton balls or a gauze sponge. Offer a towel to the patient if the face and neck are wet.	Leaving the skin moist after an irrigation is uncomfortable for the patient.
12. Remove gloves and wash your hands.	Handwashing deters the spread of microorganisms.
13. Chart the irrigation, appearance of the eye, drainage, and the patient's response.	This provides accurate documentation.

PROCEDURE 9

Administering an Ear Irrigation

Equipment

Prescribed irrigating solution (warmed to 37°C [98.6°F])
Irrigation set (container and irrigating or bulb syringe)

Emesis basin
Cotton-tipped applicators
Disposable gloves (optional)

Cotton balls
Waterproof pad

Action	Rationale
1. Explain procedure to patient.	Explanation facilitates cooperation and provides reassurance for the patient.
2. Assemble the equipment. Protect the patient and bed linens with a moisture-proof pad.	This provides for an organized approach to the task.
3. Wash your hands.	Handwashing deters the spread of microorganisms.
4. Have the patient sit up or lie with the head tilted toward the side of the affected ear. Have the patient support a basin under the ear to receive the irrigating solution.	Gravity causes the irrigating solution to flow from the ear to the basin.
5. Clean the pinna and the meatus at the auditory canal as necessary with the applicators dipped in normal saline or the irrigating solution.	Materials lodged on the pinna and at the meatus may be washed into the ear.
6. Fill the bulb syringe with solution. If an irrigating container is used, allow air to escape from the tubing.	Air forced into the ear canal is noisy and therefore unpleasant for the patient.
7. Straighten the auditory canal by pulling the pinna down and back for an infant and up and back for an adult.	Straightening the ear canal aids in allowing solution to reach all areas of the canal easily.
8. Direct a steady, slow stream of solution against the roof of the auditory canal, using only sufficient force to remove secretions. Do not occlude the auditory canal with the irrigating nozzle. Allow solution to flow out unimpeded.	Solution directed at the roof of the canal aids in preventing injury to the tympanic membrane. Continuous in-and-out flow of the irrigating solution helps to prevent pressure in the canal.

(continued)

PROCEDURE 9

Administering an Ear Irrigation (Continued)

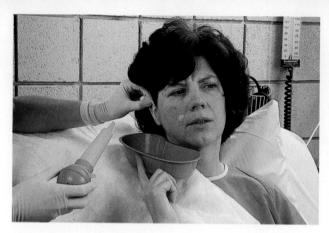

Action 7: Straightening the auditory canal.

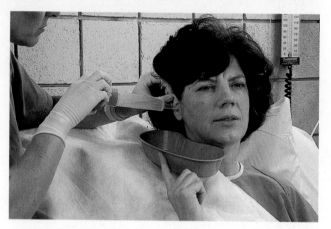

Action 8: Instilling irrigation fluid. (PHOTOS © KEN KASPER.)

9. When the irrigation is completed, place a cotton ball loosely in the auditory meatus and have the patient lie on the side of the affected ear on a towel or an absorbent pad.

The cotton ball absorbs excess fluid, and gravity allows the remaining solution in the canal to escape from the ear.

10. Wash your hands.

Handwashing deters the spread of microorganisms.

11. Chart the irrigation, the appearance of the drainage, and the patient's response.

This provides accurate documentation.

12. Return in 10 to 15 minutes and remove the cotton ball and assess drainage.

Drainage or pain may indicate injury to the tympanic membrane.

PROCEDURE 10

Starting an Intravenous Infusion

Equipment

IV solution
IV infusion set
IV tubing
IV catheter (over-the-needle, angiocath) or butterfly needle
Tourniquet
Cleansing swabs (alcohol, povidone-iodine)

Towel or disposable pad
Gauze or transparent dressing (according to agency policy)
Time tape or label (for IV container)
Site protector or tube-shaped elastic netting (optional)

Nonallergenic tape
Electronic infusion device (if ordered)
Armboard, if needed
Disposable gloves
IV pole

Action

Rationale

1. Gather all equipment and bring to bedside. Check IV solution and medication additives with physician's order.

Having equipment available saves time and facilitates accomplishment of task. Ensures that patient receives the correct IV solution and medication as ordered by physician.

2. Explain procedure to patient.

Explanation allays client's anxiety.

3. Wash your hands.

Handwashing deters the spread of microorganisms.

PROCEDURE 10

Starting an Intravenous Infusion (Continued)

4. Prepare IV solution and tubing:

   a. Maintain aseptic technique when opening sterile packages and IV solution

   b. Clamp tubing, uncap spike, and insert into entry site on bag as manufacturer directs.

   c. Squeeze drip chamber and allow it to fill at least half way.

This prevents spread of microorganisms.

This punctures the seal in the IV bag.

Suction effect causes fluid to move into drip chamber. Also prevents air from moving down the tubing.

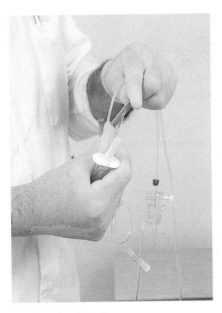
Action 4b: Clamping tubing.

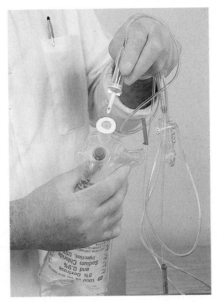
Action 4b: Inserting spike.

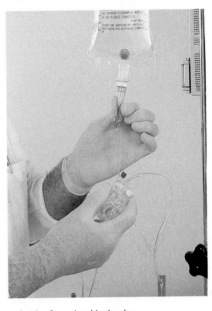
Action 4c: Squeezing drip chamber.

   d. Remove cap at end of tubing, release clamp, and allow fluid to move through tubing. Allow fluid to flow until all air bubbles have disappeared. Close clamp and recap end of tubing, maintaining sterility of setup.

This removes air from tubing that can, in larger amounts, act as an air embolus.

   e. If an electronic device is to be used, follow manufacturer's instructions for inserting tubing and setting infusion rate.

This ensures correct flow rate and proper use of equipment.

   f. Apply label if medication was added to container (pharmacy may have added medication and applied label).

This provides for administration of correct solution with prescribed medication or additive.

   g. Place time-tape on container.

This permits immediate evaluation of IV according to schedule.

5. Have the patient in a low Fowler's position in bed. Place protective towel or pad under patient's arm.

The supine position permits either arm to be used and allows for good body alignment. The low Fowler's position is usually most comfortable for the patient.

6. Select an appropriate site and palpate accessible veins.

The selection of an appropriate site decreases discomfort for the patient and possible damage to body tissues.

7. If the site is hairy and agency policy permits, clip a 2-inch area around the intended site of entry.

It is difficult to clean the site of entry in the presence of hair because hair can harbor microorganisms.

(continued)

8. Apply a tourniquet 5 to 6 inches above the venipuncture site to obstruct venous blood flow and distend the vein. Direct the ends of the tourniquet away from the site of entry. Check to be sure that the radial pulse is still present.

Interrupting the blood flow to the heart causes the vein to distend. Interruption of the arterial flow impedes venous filling. Distended veins are easy to see, palpate, and enter. The end of the tourniquet could contaminate the area of injection if directed toward the site of entry.

9. Ask the patient to open and close his or her fist. Observe and palpate for a suitable vein. Try the following techniques if a vein cannot be felt:

   a. Release the tourniquet and have the patient lower his or her arm below the level of the heart to fill the veins. Reapply tourniquet and gently tap over the intended vein to help distend it.

   b. Remove tourniquet and place warm moist compresses over the intended vein for 10 to 15 minutes.

Contraction of the muscles of the forearm forces blood into the veins, thereby distending them further. Lowering the arm below the level of the heart, tapping the vein, and applying warmth help distend veins by filling them with blood.

10. Don clean gloves.

Care must be used when handling any blood or body fluids to prevent transmission of HIV and other blood-borne infections.

11. Cleanse the entry site with an antiseptic solution (alcohol swab) followed by antimicrobial solution (povidone-iodine) according to agency policy. Use a circular motion to move from the center outward for several inches.

Cleansing that begins at the site of entry and moves outward in a circular motion carries organisms away from the site of entry. Organisms on the skin can be introduced into the tissues or the bloodstream with the needle.

12. Use the nondominant hand, placed about 1 inch or 2 inches below entry site, to hold the skin taut against the vein. Avoid touching the prepared site.

Pressure on the vein and surrounding tissues helps prevent movement of the vein as the needle or catheter is being inserted. The needle entry site and catheter must remain free of contamination from unsterile hands.

13. Enter the skin gently with the catheter held by the hub in the dominant hand, bevel side up, at a 10- to 30-degree angle. The catheter may be inserted from directly over the vein or the side of the vein. While following the course of the vein, advance the needle or catheter into the vein. A sensation of "give" can be felt when the needle enters the vein.

This allows needle or catheter to enter the vein with minimal trauma and deters passage of the needle through the vein.

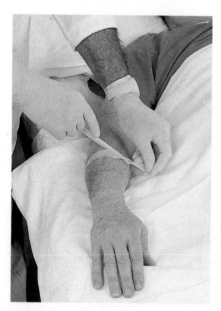

Action 8: Applying tourniquet.

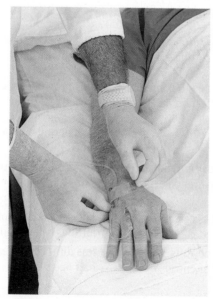

Action 18: Looping and anchoring tubing.

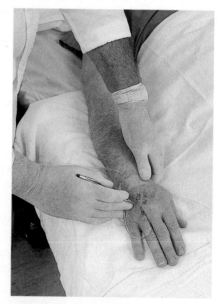

Action 19: Marking pertinent information on tape.

(PHOTOS © B. PROUD.)

PROCEDURE 10

Starting an Intravenous Infusion (Continued)

14. When blood returns through the lumen of the needle or the flashback chamber of the catheter, advance either device ⅛ to ¼ inch farther into the vein. A catheter needs to be advanced until the hub is at the venipuncture site, but the exact technique depends on the type of device used.

The tourniquet causes increased venous pressure resulting in automatic backflow. Having the catheter placed well into the vein helps to prevent dislodgement.

15. Release the tourniquet. Quickly remove protective cap from the IV tubing and attach the tubing to the catheter or needle. Stabilize the catheter or needle with nondominant hand.

Bleeding is minimized and patency of the vein is maintained if the connection is made smoothly between the catheter and tubing.

16. Start the flow of solution promptly by releasing the clamp on the tubing. Examine the tissue around the entry site for signs of infiltration.

Blood clots readily if intravenous flow is not maintained. If catheter accidentally slips out of vein, solution will accumulate and infiltrate into surrounding tissue.

17. Secure the catheter with narrow nonallergenic tape (½ inch) placed sticky side up under the hub and crossed over the top of the hub.

The smooth structure of the vein does not offer resistance to the movement of the catheter. The weight of the tubing is sufficient to pull it out of the vein if it is not well anchored. Nonallergenic tape is less likely to tear fragile skin.

18. Place sterile dressing over venipuncture site. Agency policy may direct nurse to use gauze dressing or transparent dressing. Apply tape to dressing if necessary. Loop the tubing near the site of entry, and anchor to dressing.

Transparent dressing allows easy visualization of site but may place patient at increased risk for infection. Gauze dressing absorbs drainage and may have a decreased infection rate. Discussion continues about effectiveness of types of dressings.

19. Mark the date, time, site and type and size of the catheter used for the infusion on the tape anchoring the tubing.

Personnel working with the infusion will know what type of device is being used, the site, and when it was inserted. Protects patient and IV site from infection.

20. Anchor arm to an armboard for support if necessary or apply a site protector or tube-shaped mesh netting over the insertion site.

An armboard or site protectors help to prevent change in the position of the catheter in the vein.

21. Adjust the rate of solution flow according to the amount prescribed or follow manufacturer's directions for adjusting flow rate on infusion pump.

The physician prescribes the rate of flow.

22. Remove all equipment and dispose in proper manner. Remove gloves and wash hands.

Handwashing deters the spread of microorganisms.

23. Document the procedure and patient's response. Chart time, site, device used, and solution.

This provides accurate documentation and ensures continuity of care.

24. Return to check flow rate and observe for infiltration 30 minutes after starting infusion.

This documents patient's response to infusion.

Age Considerations

- *Older adults:* Avoid vigorous friction at the insertion site and using too much alcohol. Both can traumatize fragile skin and veins in the elderly (Roth, 1997).
- Experienced nurses may elect to omit use of a tourniquet on individuals with prominent but especially fragile veins. This decreases trauma to the vessel.
- *Children:* Hand insertion sites should not be the first choice for children because nerve endings are very close to the surface of the skin and it is more painful. Research indicates that peripheral IVs should not remain in place longer than 6 days for children or the risk for infection increases. Adults have a 2- to 3-day limit because they are at risk for developing phlebitis, which is rarely seen in children (Frey, 1998).

PROCEDURE 11

Changing IV Solution and Tubing

Equipment

For solution change:
  IV solution as ordered
    by physician

For tubing change:
  Administration set
  Sterile gauze
  Timing tape or label

Sterile dressings and antiseptic
  solutions (according to agency
  recommendations)
Disposable gloves

Action	Rationale
1. Gather all equipment and bring to bedside. Check IV solution and medication additives with physician's order.	Having equipment available saves time and facilitates accomplishment of task. Ensures that patient receives the correct IV solution and medication as ordered by physician.
2. Explain procedure to patient.	Explanation allays patient's anxiety.
3. Wash your hands.	Handwashing deters the spread of microorganisms.

To Change IV Solution

Action	Rationale
4. Carefully remove protective cover from new solution container and expose entry site.	This maintains sterility of IV solution.
5. Close clamp on tubing.	Clamping stops the flow of IV fluid during change of solution.
6. Lift container off IV pole and invert it. Quickly remove the spike from the old IV container, being careful not to contaminate it.	This maintains sterility of IV setup.
7. Steady new container and insert spike. Hang on IV pole.	This allows for uninterrupted flow of new solution.
8. Reopen clamp on tubing and adjust flow.	Opening clamp regulates flow rate into drip chamber.
9. Label container according to agency policy. Record on intake and output record and document on chart according to agency policy. Discard used equipment in proper manner. Wash your hands.	This ensures accurate continuation and administration of correct IV solution. Handwashing deters the spread of microorganisms.

To Change IV Tubing and Solution

Action	Rationale
10. Follow actions 1 through 4.	This maintains sterility of IV setup. Once clamp is closed, the bag can be spiked without loss of solution.
11. Open the administration set and close clamp on new tubing. Remove protective covering from infusion spike. Using sterile technique, insert into new container.	
12. Hang IV container on pole and squeeze drip chamber to fill at least halfway.	Gravity and suction effect cause fluid to move into drip chamber.
13. Remove cap at end of tubing, release clamp, and allow fluid to move through tubing until all air bubbles have disappeared. Close clamp and recap end of tubing maintaining sterility of setup.	This removes air from tubing that can, in larger amounts, act as an air embolus.
14. Loosen tape at IV insertion site. Don clean gloves. Carefully remove dressing and tape.	Care must be used when blood contact is possible. This prevents transmission of HIV and other blood-borne infections. Removing dressing provides access to needle hub necessary for tubing change.

PROCEDURE 11

Changing IV Solution and Tubing (Continued)

15. Place sterile gauze square under needle hub.

Gauze absorbs any leakage when tubing is disconnected from needle.

16. Place new IV tubing close to patient's IV site and slightly loosen protective cap.

This facilitates removal of cap and attachment to needle hub.

17. Clamp the old IV tubing. Steady the needle hub with nondominant hand until change is completed. Remove tubing with dominant hand using a twisting motion. A short closed tubing set with an injection port and closure clamp between the needle or angiocath hub and the tubing may also be used.

This stabilizes needle and prevents inadvertently dislodging it. The use of a short closed tubing set reduces risk for blood exposure.

18. Set old tubing aside. While maintaining sterility, carefully remove cap and insert sterile end of tubing into the needle hub. Twist to secure it. Remove soiled gloves.

This maintains sterility of IV setup.

19. Open the clamp.

Opening clamp allows solution to flow to patient.

20. Reapply sterile dressing to site according to agency protocol (see Procedure 13).

This deters entry of microorganisms at site.

21. Regulate the IV flow according to physician's order.

This ensures that patient receives IV solution at the prescribed rate.

22. Attach to IV tubing tape or label (see photo) that states date, time, and your initials. Label container and record procedure (see photo) according to agency policy. Discard used equipment in proper manner and wash hands.

This documents IV tubing change. Handwashing deters the spread of microorganisms.

23. Record patient's response to IV infusion.

This ensures accurate documentation of patient's response.

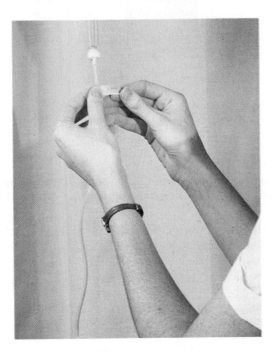

Action 22: Labeling IV tubing.

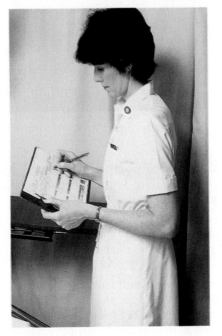

Action 23: Recording patient's response to infusion.

Monitoring an IV Site and Infusion

Action	**Rationale**
1. Monitor IV infusion several times a shift. More frequent checks may be necessary if medication is being infused:	This promotes safe administration of IV fluids and medication. Too rapid administration of medications can result in the development of speed shock.
a. Check physician's order for IV solution.	This ensures that correct solution is being given at the correct rate and in the proper sequence with the correct medications.
b. Check drip chamber and time drops (see photo) if IV is not regulated by an infusion control device.	This ensures that flow rate is correct.
c. Check tubing for anything that might interfere with flow. Be sure that clamp is in the open position. Observe dressing for leakage of IV solution.	Any kink or pressure on tubing may interfere with flow. Leakage may occur at connection of tubing with hub of needle or catheter and allow for loss of IV solution.

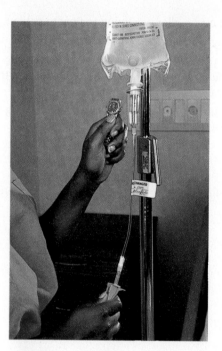

Action 1b: Timing the drops.

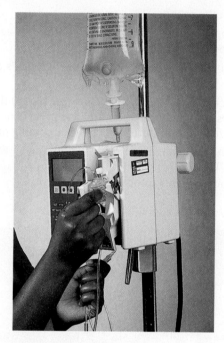

Action 1d: Setting up the pump.

d. Observe settings, alarm, and indicator lights on infusion control device if one is being used (see photo).	Observation ensures that infusion control device is functioning and that alarm is in ON position.
2. Inspect site for swelling, pain, coolness, or pallor at site of insertion, which may indicate infiltration of IV. This necessitates removing IV and restarting at another site.	Catheter may become dislodged from vein, and IV solution may flow into subcutaneous tissue.
3. Inspect site (see photo) for redness, swelling, heat, and pain at the IV site, which may indicate phlebitis is present. IV will need to be discontinued and restarted at another site. Notify physician if you suspect that phlebitis may have occurred.	Chemical irritation or mechanical trauma cause injury to the vein and can lead to the development of phlebitis.

PROCEDURE 12

Monitoring an IV Site and Infusion (Continued)

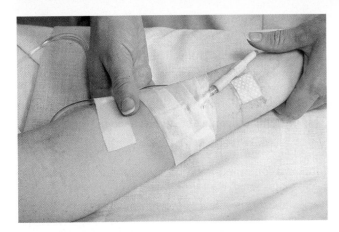

Action 3: Checking inflammation surrounding infusion site. (PHOTOS © B. PROUD.)

4. Check for local or systemic manifestations that indicate an infection is present at the site. IV will be discontinued and physician notified. Be careful not to disconnect IV tubing when putting on patient's hospital gown.

Poor aseptic technique may allow bacteria to enter the needle or catheter insertion site or tubing connection.

5. Be alert for additional complications of IV therapy.
   a. Circulatory overload can result in signs of cardiac failure and pulmonary edema. Monitor intake and output during IV therapy.
   b. Bleeding at the site is most likely to occur when the IV is discontinued.

Infusing too much IV solution results in an increased volume of circulating fluid.

Bleeding may be caused by anticoagulant medication.

6. If possible, instruct patient to call for assistance if any discomfort is noted at site, solution container is nearly empty, or flow has changed in any way.

This facilitates cooperation of patient and safe administration of IV solution.

7. Document IV infusion, any complications of therapy, and patient's reaction to therapy.

This provides accurate documentation and ensures continuity of care.

PROCEDURE 13

Changing an IV Dressing

Equipment

Sterile gauze (2 × 2 or 4 × 4) or
    transparent occlusive dressing
Povidone-iodine (Betadine) swabs
Adhesive remover (optional)

Alcohol swabs
Tape
Clean gloves

Towel or disposable pad
Masks for nurse and patient
    (optional)

Action

Rationale

Peripheral

1. Assess patient's need for dressing change.

Agency policy determines interval for dressing change (every 24 to 72 hours). The presence of moisture or a nonadhering dressing increases risk for bacterial contamination at the site.

(continued)

Changing an IV Dressing (Continued)

2. Gather equipment and bring to bedside. Place towel or disposable pad under extremity.

Having equipment available saves time and facilitates the performance of the task.

3. Explain procedure to patient.

Explanation allays patient's anxiety.

4. Wash your hands. Don clean gloves.

Handwashing deters the spread of microorganisms. Gloves prevent transmission of HIV and other blood-borne infections.

5. Carefully remove old dressing but leave tape that anchors IV needle or catheter in place. Discard in proper manner.

This prevents dislodging of IV needle or catheter.

6. Assess IV site for presence of inflammation or infiltration. Discontinue and relocate the IV if noted.

Inflammation or infiltration causes trauma to tissues and necessitates removal of the IV needle or catheter.

7. Loosen tape and gently remove, being careful to steady catheter with one hand. Use adhesive remover if necessary.

Tape stabilizes needle and prevents inadvertently dislodging it.

8. Cleanse the entry site with an alcohol swab using a circular motion moving from the center outward. Allow to dry. Follow with povidone-iodine swab using the same process.

Cleaning in a circular motion while moving outward carries organisms away from the entry site. Use of antiseptic solutions reduces the number of microorganisms on the skin surface.

9. Reapply tape strip to needle or catheter at entry site.

Tape anchors needle or catheter to prevent dislodgement.

10. Apply sterile gauze or transparent polyurethane dressing over entry site. Remove gloves and dispose of properly.

Dressing protects site and deters contamination with microorganisms.

11. Secure IV tubing with additional tape if necessary. Label dressing with date, time of change, and initials. Check that IV flow is accurate and system is patent.

Label documents IV dressing change.

Central Venous Access Device

12. Follow Actions 1–5.

13. Remove gloves and wash hands thoroughly. If agency requires, nurse and patient should put on a mask. Open dressing kit using sterile technique.

Unclean hands and improper technique are potential sources for infecting a central venous access device. Most facilities have all sterile dressing supplies gathered in a single unit.

14. Put on sterile gloves.

Maintains surgical asepsis.

15. Using the alcohol swabs, move in a circular fashion from the insertion site outward (1½- to 2-inch area). Allow to dry.

The alcohol kills *Staphylococcus aureus* and *epidermis*, which are the most common causes of central line infections (Masoorli, 1997).

16. Follow alcohol cleansing with povidone-iodine swabs using the same technique. Allow to dry.

Povidone-iodine kills fungi that are responsible for 25% of central line infections (Masoorli, 1997c).

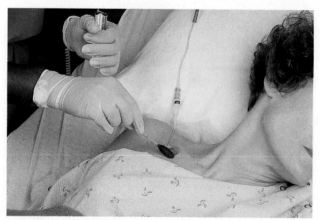

Action 16: Cleaning with povidone-iodine swabs.

PROCEDURE 13

Changing an IV Dressing (Continued)

17. Reapply sterile dressing or securement device according to agency policy. Secure tubing or lumens to prevent tugging on insertion site.

Prevents contamination of the IV catheter and protects insertion site.

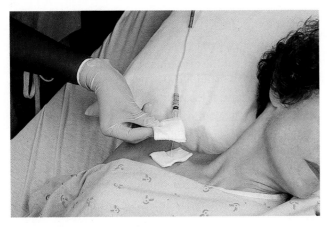

Action 17: Applying a sterile dressing.

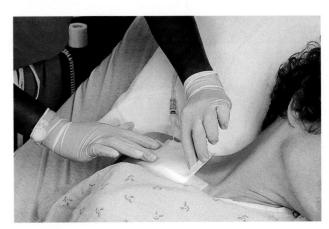

Action 17: Securing the dressing with tape.

18. Note date, time of dressing change, size of catheter, and initials on tape or dressing.

Documents that dressing change occurred.

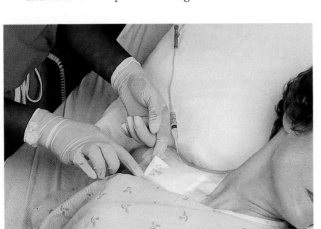

Action 18: Labeling the dressing.

19. Discard equipment properly and wash hands.

20. Record patient's response to dressing change and observation of site.

Handwashing protects against spread of microorganisms.

This provides accurate documentation and ensures continuity of care.

PROCEDURE 14

Capping a Primary Line for Intermittent Use

Equipment

Lock device
Clean gloves
4 × 4 gauze pad

Normal saline or heparin flush
  prepared in a syringe (1–3 mL)
  according to agency policy

Alcohol wipe
Tape
Extension tubing (optional)

Action	Rationale
1. Gather equipment and verify physician's order. Fill lock and extension tubing with normal saline or heparin flush. Recap syringe for use in number 10.	Having equipment available saves time and facilitates the task; ensures that the procedure has been ordered by the physician. Flush maintains patency of lock and tubing.
2. Explain the procedure to the patient.	Explanation allays the patient's anxiety.
3. Wash your hands.	Handwashing deters the spread of microorganisms.
4. Assess the IV site.	Complications such as infiltration or phlebitis necessitate discontinuation of the IV infusion at that site.
5. Clamp off primary line.	Protects patient and nurse from inadvertent blood loss when IV and tubing are disconnected.
6. Don clean gloves.	Gloves protect the nurse from contact with the patient's blood.
7. Place gauze 4 × 4 sponge underneath IV connection hub between IV catheter and tubing.	Gauze absorbs any blood leakage when IV and tubing are disconnected.
8. Stabilize hub of IV catheter with nondominant hand. Use dominant hand to quickly twist and disconnect IV tubing from the catheter, discard it, and attach prefilled lock device or needleless cap to hub without contaminating the tips of the catheter and lock. Extension tubing may also be attached.	This maintains sterility of IV setup.

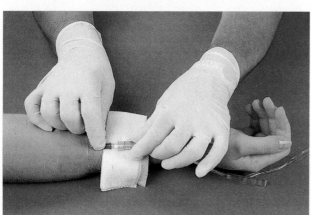

Action 8: Disconnecting tubing from an IV catheter.

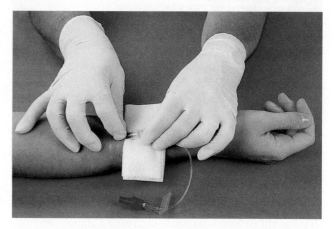

Action 8: Attaching a lock device with extension tubing to the IV catheter hub.

9. Cleanse cap with an alcohol wipe.	Cleansing removes surface bacteria at the heparin lock entry site.
10. Insert the syringe with blunt cannula or standard syringe and gently flush catheter with saline or heparin flush as per agency policy. Remove syringe carefully.	This maintains patency of the IV access line. Clinical evidence has demonstrated that a saline flush is as effective as heparin for peripheral IVs and avoids the adverse effects of heparin, is less expensive, and prevents drug incompatibilities.
11. Tape lock or cap securely in place.	Tape secures the lock and IV in place.
12. Chart on IV administration record or medication Kardex per institutional policy.	Accurate documentation is necessary to prevent error.

Adding Medications to an IV Solution Container

Equipment

Medication prepared in a syringe
with a 19- to 21-gauge needle
(or needleless device)

Alcohol swab
IV fluid container (bag or bottle)

Label to be attached to the IV
container

Action	**Rationale**
1. Gather all equipment and bring to the patient's bedside. Check the medication order with the physician's order.	Having equipment available saves time and facilitates performance of the task. Checking the orders ensures that the patient receives the correct medication at the correct time and in the right manner.
2. Explain the procedure to the patient.	Explanation allays the patient's anxiety.
3. Wash your hands.	Handwashing deters the spread of microorganisms.
4. Identify the patient by checking the band on the patient's wrist and asking the patient his or her name.	This ensures that medication is given to the right person.
5. Add the medication to the IV solution that is infusing:	
a. Check that the volume in the bag or bottle is adequate.	The volume should be sufficient to dilute the drug.
b. Close the IV clamp.	This prevents back-flow directly to the patient of improperly diluted medication.
c. Clean the medication port with an alcohol swab.	This deters entry of microorganisms when the needle punctures the port.
d. Steady the container and uncap the needle or needleless device and insert it into the port. Inject the medication.	This ensures that the needle or needleless device enters the container and medication can be dispersed into the solution.
e. Remove the container from the IV pole and gently rotate the solutions.	This mixes the medication with the solution.

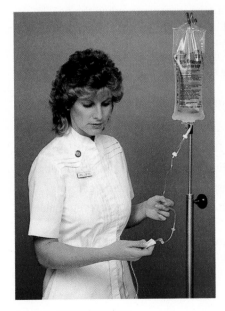

Action 5b: Closing the IV clamp.

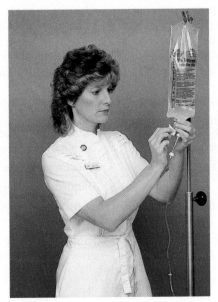

Action 5c: Cleaning the medication port.

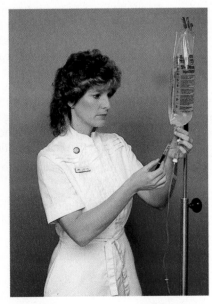

Action 5d: Inserting the needle or needleless device into the port.

(continued)

PROCEDURE 15

Adding Medications to an IV Solution Container (Continued)

f. Rehang the container, open the clamp, and readjust the flow rate.

g. Attach the label to the container so that the dose of medication that has been added is apparent.

This ensures the infusion of the IV with medication at the prescribed rate.

This confirms that the prescribed dose of medication has been added to the IV solution.

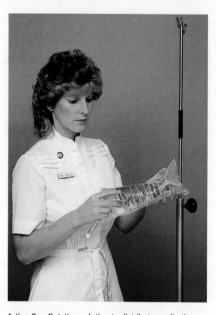

Action 5e: Rotating solution to distribute medication.

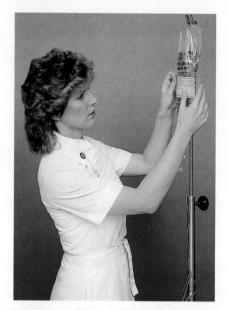

Action 5g: Labeling container to show medication.

(PHOTOS © KEN KASPER.)

6. Add the medication to the IV solution before infusion:

a. Carefully remove any protective cover and locate the injection port. Clean with an alcohol swab.

b. Uncap the needle or needleless device and insert into the port. Inject the medication.

c. Withdraw and insert the spike into the proper entry site on the bag or bottle.

d. With tubing clamped, gently rotate the IV solution in the bag or bottle. Hang the IV.

e. Attach the label to the container so that the dose of medication that has been added is apparent.

7. Dispose of equipment according to agency policy.

8. Wash your hands.

9. Chart the addition of medication to the IV solution.

10. Evaluate the patient's response to medication within the appropriate time frame.

This deters entry of microorganisms when the needle punctures the port.

This ensures that the needle enters the container and that medication can be dispersed into the solution.

This punctures the seal in the IV bag or bottle.

This mixes medication with the solution.

This confirms that the prescribed dose of medication has been added to the IV solution.

This prevents inadvertent injury from the equipment.

Handwashing deters the spread of microorganisms.

Accurate documentation is necessary to prevent medication errors.

Patients require careful observation because medications given by the IV route may have a rapid effect.

PROCEDURE 16

Adding a Bolus IV Medication to an Existing IV

Equipment

Medication prepared in a syringe
    with needleless device or 23- to
    25-gauge, 1-inch needle

Alcohol swab
Watch with second hand
Disposable gloves

Action	Rationale
1. Gather the equipment and bring to the patient's bedside. Check the medication order with the physician's order. Check a drug resource to clarify if medication needs to be diluted before administration.	Having equipment available saves time and facilitates performance of the task. Checking the orders ensures that the patient receives the correct medication at the correct time and in the right manner.
2. Explain the procedure to the patient.	Explanation allays the patient's anxiety.
3. Wash your hands. Don clean gloves.	Handwashing deters the spread of microorganisms. Gloves protect the nurse from exposure to blood-borne pathogens.
4. Identify the patient by checking the band on the patient's wrist and asking the patient his or her name.	This ensures that medication is given to the right person.
5. Assess the IV site for the presence of inflammation or infiltration.	IV medication must be given directly into a vein for safe administration.
6. Select the injection port on the tubing that is closest to the venipuncture site. Clean the port with an alcohol swab.	Using the port closest to the needle insertion site minimizes dilution of the medication. Cleaning with alcohol deters entry of microorganisms when the needle punctures the port.
7. Uncap the syringe. Steady the port with your nondominant hand while inserting the needleless device or needle into the center of the port.	This supports the injection port and lessens the risk for accidentally dislodging the IV or entering the port incorrectly.
8. Move your nondominant hand to the section of IV tubing just beyond the injection port. Fold the tubing between your fingers to temporarily stop the flow of the IV solution.	This minimizes the dilution of the IV medication with IV solution.
9. Pull back slightly on the plunger just until blood appears in the tubing.	This ensures injection of medication into a vein.

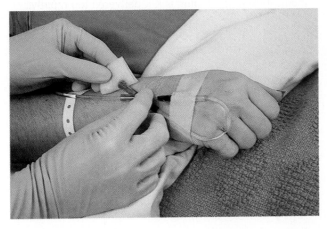

Action 6: Cleaning injection port.

(continued)

PROCEDURE 16

Adding a Bolus IV Medication to an Existing IV (Continued)

10. Inject the medication at the prescribed rate. (see Special Considerations, below).

This delivers the correct amount of medication at the proper interval according to manufacturer's directions.

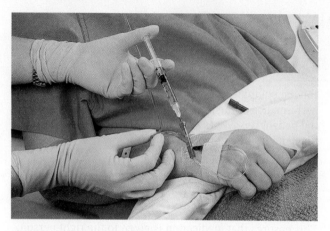

Action 10: Injecting medication while interrupting IV flow. (PHOTO © B. PROUD)

11. Remove the needle. Do not cap it. Release the tubing and allow the IV to flow at the proper rate.

This prevents accidental needlestick.

12. Dispose of the syringe in the proper receptacle.

Proper disposal prevents accidental injury and spread of microorganisms.

13. Remove gloves and wash your hands.

Handwashing deters the spread of microorganisms.

14. Chart the administration of the medication.

Accurate documentation is necessary to prevent medication errors.

15. Evaluate the patient's response to medication within the appropriate time frame.

The patient requires careful observation because medications given by an IV bolus injection may have a rapid effect.

Special Considerations

Agency policy may recommend the following variations when injecting a bolus IV medication:

- Release the folded tubing after a portion of the drug has been administered at the prescribed rate to facilitate delivery of the medication.
- Use a syringe with 1 mL normal saline to flush the tubing after an IV bolus is delivered to ensure that residual medication in the tubing is not delivered too rapidly.

Administering IV Medications by Piggyback, Volume-Control Administration Set, or Miniinfusion Pump

Equipment

For Piggyback or Miniinfusion Pump

Gloves (optional)
Medication prepared in labeled
  piggyback set or syringe
  (5 to 100 mL)
Secondary infusion tubing (microdrip
  or macrodrip)
Needleless device, stopcock, or sterile
  needle (21- to 23-gauge)
Alcohol swab
Tape
Metal or plastic hook
Miniinfusion pump
Date label for tubing

For Volume Control Set

Gloves (optional)
Volume-control set (eg, Volutrol,
  Buretrol)
Medication (in vial or ampule)
Syringe with needleless device
  attached or a 20- or 21-gauge
  needle
Alcohol swab
Medication label

Action	Rationale
1. Gather all equipment and bring to the patient's bedside. Check the medication order against the original physician's order according to agency policy.	Having equipment available saves time and facilitates performance of the task. Checking the orders ensures that the patient receives the correct medication at the correct time and in the right manner.
2. Identify the patient by checking the identification band on the patient's wrist and asking the patient his or her name.	This ensures that the medication is given to the right person.
3. Explain the procedure to the patient.	Explanation allays the patient's anxiety.
4. Wash your hands and don gloves.	Handwashing deters the spread of microorganisms. Gloves protect the nurse when connecting setup to an existing IV.
5. Assess the IV site for the presence of inflammation or infiltration.	The medication must be administered directly into the vein that is not inflamed to avoid injuring surrounding tissue.

For Piggyback Infusion

Action	Rationale
6. Attach the infusion tubing to the piggyback set containing diluted medication. Place label on tubing with appropriate date and attach needle or needleless device to end of tubing according to manufacturer's directions. Open the clamp and prime the tubing (see action 4, Procedure 10). Close the clamp.	This removes air from the tubing and preserves the sterility of the setup. Tubing for piggyback setup may be used for 48 to 72 hours, depending on agency policy.
7. Hang the piggyback container on the IV pole, positioning it higher than the primary IV according to the manufacturer's recommendations. Use metal or plastic hook to lower primary IV.	The position of the container influences the flow of the IV fluid into the primary setup.
8. Use an alcohol swab to clean the appropriate port.	This deters entry of microorganisms when the piggyback setup is connected to the port.

9. Connect the piggyback setup to either:
  a. Needleless port
  b. Stopcock: turn stopcock to open position
	Needleless systems and stopcock setup eliminate the need for a needle and are recommended by the Centers for Disease Control and Prevention.

(continued)

c. Primary IV line: uncap needle and insert into secondary IV port closest to the top of the primary tubing. Use a strip of tape to secure the secondary set tubing to the primary infusion tubing. Primary line is left unclamped if port has a back-flow valve.

The tape stabilizes the needle in the infusion port and prevents it from slipping out. Back-flow valve in primary line secondary port stops flow of primary infusion while piggyback solution is infusing. Once completed, the back-flow valve opens, and flow of primary solution resumes.

10. Open the clamp on the piggyback set and regulate the flow at the prescribed delivery rate or set rate for secondary infusion on infusion pump. Monitor the medication infusion at periodic intervals.

Delivery over a 30- to 60-minute interval is usually a safe method of administering IV medication. It is important to verify safe administration rate for each drug to prevent adverse effects.

11. Clamp the tubing on the piggyback set when the solution is infused. Follow agency policy regarding disposal of equipment.

This reduces the risk for contaminating the primary IV setup.

12. Readjust the flow rate of the primary IV.

Piggyback medication administration may interrupt the normal flow rate of the primary IV. Readjustment of the rate may be necessary.

Using a Miniinfusion Pump

13. Connect prepared syringe to miniinfusion tubing.

Special tubing connects prepared medication to primary IV line.

14. Fill tubing with medication by applying gentle pressure to syringe plunger.

This removes air from the tubing.

15. Insert syringe into miniinfusion pump according to manufacturer's directions.

Syringe must fit securely in pump apparatus for proper operation.

16. Connect miniinfusion tubing to appropriate connector as in action 9.

Proper connection allows IV medication to flow into primary IV line.

17. Program pump to begin infusion. Set alarm if recommended by manufacturer.

Pump delivers medication at controlled rate. Alarm is recommended for use with IV lock apparatus.

18. Recheck flow rate of primary IV once pump has completed delivery of medication.

Normal flow rate of the primary IV may have been altered by the miniinfusion pump.

Using a Volume-Control Administration Set

19. Withdraw medication from the vial or ampule into the prepared syringe. See Procedure 1 or 2.

The correct dose is prepared for dilution in the IV solution.

20. Open the clamp between the IV solution and the volume-control administration set or secondary setup. Follow the manufacturer's instructions and fill with the desired amount of IV solution. Close the clamp.

This dilutes the medication in the minimal amount of solution. Reclamping prevents the continued addition of fluid to the volume to be mixed with the medication.

21. Use an alcohol swab to clean the injection port on the secondary setup.

This deters entry of microorganisms when the needle punctures the port.

22. Remove the cap and insert the needle or blunt needleless device into the port while holding the syringe steady. Inject the medication. Mix gently with IV solution.

This ensures that the medication is evenly mixed with solution.

23. Open the clamp below the secondary setup and regulate at the prescribed delivery rate. Monitor the medication infusion at periodic intervals.

Delivery over a 30- to 60-minute interval is a safe method of administering IV medication.

24. Attach the label to the volume-control device.

This prevents medication error.

25. Place the syringe with the uncapped needle in the designated container.

Proper disposal of the needle prevents inadvertent needlestick.

Administering IV Medications by Piggyback, Volume-Control Administration Set, or Miniinfusion Pump (Continued)

26. Wash your hands.

27. Chart the administration of medication after it has been infused.

28. Evaluate the patient's response to medication within the appropriate time frame.

Handwashing deters the spread of microorganisms.

Accurate documentation is necessary to prevent medication errors.

The patient requires careful observation because medications given by the IV route may have a rapid effect.

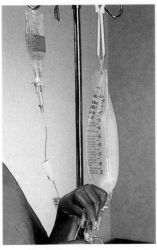

Action 6: Attaching tubing to piggyback set.

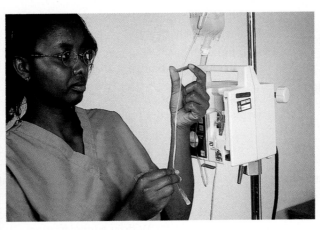

Action 6: Opening clamp and priming the tube.

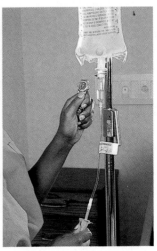

Action 9a: Connecting piggyback setup to needleless port.

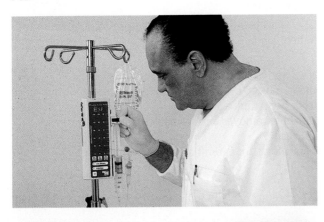

Action 15: Inserting syringe into mini-infusion pump.

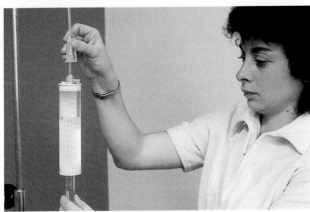

Action 20: Filling volume-control set.

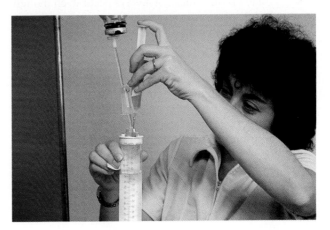

Action 22: Injecting medication.

Introducing Drugs Through a Heparin or Intravenous Lock Using the Saline Flush

Equipment

Medication
Medication Kardex or computer-
    generated MAR
Saline vial
Sterile syringe (2) with needleless
    device or 25-gauge needle
Alcohol swabs
Watch with second hand or digital
    readout
Gloves

For Bolus Injection
Sterile syringe (2) with needleless
    device or 25-gauge needle

For Intermittent IV Delivery
IV setup with needleless device
    attached to tubing or a 25-gauge
    needle
Adhesive tape (optional)
IV pump or controller (optional)

Action	Rationale
1. Assemble the equipment and check the physician's order.	This ensures that the patient receives the right medication at the right time by the proper route.
2. Explain the procedure to the patient.	Explanation alleviates the patient's apprehension about IV drug administration.
3. Wash your hands.	Handwashing deters the spread of microorganisms.
4. Withdraw 1 to 2 mL of sterile saline from the vial into the syringe as described in Procedure 2.	Using saline eliminates concern about drug incompatibilities and effect on systemic circulation that exists with heparin flush.
5. Don the clean gloves.	Gloves protect the nurse's hands from contact with the patient's blood.
6. Administer the medication. *For bolus IV injection:*	
a. Check the drug package for the correct injection rate for the IV push route.	Using the correct injection rate prevents speed shock from occurring.
b. Clean the port of the lock with an alcohol swab.	Cleaning removes surface bacteria at the heparin lock entry site.
c. Stabilize the port with your nondominant hand and insert the needleless device or needle of syringe of normal saline into the port.	This allows for careful insertion into the center circle of the lock.
d. Aspirate gently and check for blood return (blood return does not always occur even though lock is patent).	Blood return usually indicates that the catheter is in vein.
e. Gently flush with 1 mL of normal saline. Remove the syringe.	Saline flush ensures that the IV line is patent. A patient's complaint of pain or resistance to the flush detected by the nurse may indicate that the IV line is not patent.
f. Insert blunt needleless device or needle of syringe with medication into port and gently inject the medication, using a watch to verify correct injection rate. Do not force the injection if resistance is felt. If the lock is clogged, it has to be changed. Remove the medication syringe and needle when administration is completed.	Easy instillation of the medication usually indicates that the lock is still patent and in the vein. If force is used against resistance, a clot may break away and cause a blockage somewhere else in the body.

Introducing Drugs Through a Heparin or Intravenous Lock Using the Saline Flush (Continued)

For administration of a drug by way of an intermittent delivery system:

    a. Use a drug resource book to check for the correct flow rate of the medication. (The usual rate is 30 to 60 minutes.)

Using the correct injection rate prevents speed shock from occurring.

    b. Connect the infusion tubing to the medication setup according to the manufacturer's directions. Hang the IV setup on a pole. Open clamp and allow solution to clear IV tubing of air. Reclamp tubing.

This removes air from the tubing and preserves the sterility of the setup.

    c. Attach needleless connector or sterile 25-gauge needle to the end of the infusion tubing.

A small-gauge needle prevents damage to the lock.

    d. Clean the port of the lock with an alcohol swab.

Cleaning removes surface bacteria at the lock entry site. This allows for careful insertion into the port.

    e. Stabilize the port with your nondominant hand and insert the needleless device or needle of syringe of normal saline into the port.

    f. Aspirate gently and check for blood return (blood return does not always occur even though lock is patent).

Blood return usually indicates that the catheter is in vein.

    g. Gently flush with 1 mL of normal saline. Remove the syringe.

Saline flush ensures that the IV line is patent.

    h. Insert blunt needleless device or needle attached to tubing into port. If necessary, secure with tape.

Tape secures the needle in the lock port.

    i. Open the clamp and regulate the flow rate or attach to IV pump or controller according to manufacturer's directions. Close clamp when infusion is complete.

This ensures that the patient receives the medication at the correct rate.

    j. Remove the needleless connector or needle from lock. Carefully replace uncapped, used needle or needleless device with a new sterile one. Allow the medication setup to hang on the pole for future use according to agency policy. Stabilize the port with your nondominant hand and insert the needleless device or needle of syringe of normal saline into the port. Flush the reservoir with 1 to 2 mL of sterile saline. Remove the syringe and discard uncapped needles and syringes in the appropriate receptacle. Remove gloves and discard appropriately.

This prevents possible needlestick with contaminated needle. Agency policy specifies length of time for safe use of IV infusion tubing.

Saline clears the line of medication with less of the systemic effects of the heparin flush.

7. Wash your hands.

Handwashing deters the spread of microorganisms.

8. The injection site and IV lock should be checked at least every 8 hours and a small amount of saline administered if medication is not given at least that often.

This ensures the patency of the system for continuing injections.

9. The heparin lock should be changed at least every 48 hours or according to agency policy. A clogged lock should be changed immediately.

Changing a heparin lock regularly and having it free of clotted blood reduces dangers of infection and emboli in the circulating blood.

10. Chart the administration of the medication or saline flush.

Accurate documentation is necessary to prevent medication error.

(continued)

PROCEDURE 18

Introducing Drugs Through a Heparin or Intravenous Lock Using the Saline Flush (Continued)

Safety Considerations   Some agencies recommend the use of single-dose saline vials without preservatives in the solution. Preservatives may be linked to an increased incidence of phlebitis with heparin locks.

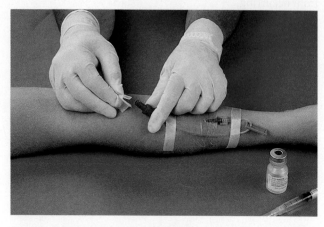

Action 6b: Cleaning the port with an alcohol swab.

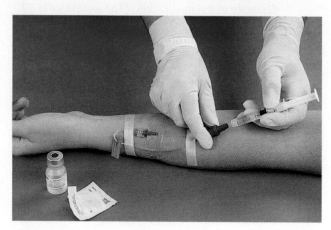

Action 6c: Inserting syringe with blunt needle into port.

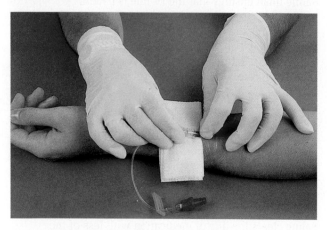

Action 6d: Aspirating for a blood return.

Appendix A
Common Types of Drug Preparations

Preparation	Description
Capsule	Powder or gel form of an active drug enclosed in a gelatinous container
Elixir	Medication in a clear liquid containing water, alcohol, sweeteners, and flavor
Extended release	Preparation of a medication that allows for slow and continuous release over a predetermined period; may also be referred to as CR or CRT (controlled release), SR (sustained or slow release), SA (sustained action), LA (long acting), or TR (timed release)
Liniment	Medication mixed with alcohol, oil, or soap, which is rubbed on the skin
Lotion	Drug particles in a solution for topical use
Lozenge	Small oval, round, or oblong preparation containing a drug in a flavored or sweetened base, which dissolves in the mouth and releases the medication; also called *troche*
Ointment	Semisolid preparation containing a drug to be applied externally; also called an *unction*
Pill	Mixture of a powdered drug with a cohesive material; may be round or oval
Powder	Single or mixture of finely ground drugs
Solution	A drug dissolved in another substance (eg, in an aqueous solution)
Suppository	An easily melted medication preparation in a firm base such as gelatin that is inserted into the body (rectum, vagina, urethra)
Suspension	Finely divided, undissolved particles in a liquid medium; should be shaken before use
Syrup	Medication combined in a water and sugar solution
Tablet	Small, solid dose of medication, compressed or molded; may be any color, size, or shape; *enteric-coated tablets* are coated with a substance that is insoluble in gastric acids to reduce gastric irritation by the drug
Transdermal patch	Unit dose of medication applied directly to skin for diffusion through skin and absorption into the bloodstream

Appendix B
Routes for Administering Drugs

Terms Used to Describe Route	How Drug Is Administered
Oral route	Having patient swallow drug
Enteral route	Administering drug through an enteral tube
Sublingual administration	Placing drug under tongue
Buccal administration	Placing drug between cheek and gum
Parenteral route	Injecting drug into
Subcutaneous injection	Subcutaneous tissue
Intramuscular injection	Muscle tissue
Intradermal injection	Corium (under epidermis)
Intravenous injection	Vein
Intraarterial injection	Artery
Intracardial injection	Heart tissue
Intraperitoneal injection	Peritoneal cavity
Intraspinal injection	Spinal canal
Intraosseous injection	Bone
Topical route	Inserting drug into
Vaginal administration	Vagina
Rectal administration	Rectum
Inunction	Rubbing drug into skin
Instillation	Placing drug into direct contact with mucous membrane
Irrigation	Flushing mucous membrane with drug in solution
Skin application	Applying transdermal patch
Pulmonary route	Having patient inhale drug

Appendix C
Assessment Guide

Medications

Factors to Assess	Questions and Approaches
Previous and current drug use	What medications are you taking that the doctor prescribed for you?
	What over-the-counter medications are you taking on a regular basis?
	Do you use nonmedicinal drugs (eg, alcohol, caffeine, home remedies)?
	How often do you use them?
	What is the reason for taking the medication?
	What medications have you taken during the past year and for what reasons?
	Is there anything else you have tried to alleviate your symptoms?
Medication schedule	At what times do you take your medications?
	Is there any special way your medication has to be prepared (eg, crushing and mixing with applesauce)?
	Do you have any special method for remembering to take your medications?
Response to medications	Have the medications had the expected effects?
	Have you ever experienced any adverse or unexpected reactions to the medications?
	Is there a family history of this type of reaction to medication?
	Do you have any allergies to medications?
	What happens when you take this medication?
Attitude toward drugs and use of drugs	How do you feel about taking medications?
	Why do you take the medications?
Compliance with regimen	Can you tell me your understanding of the reason for taking the medications?
	Can you describe how you follow the medication schedule?
	Are there any problems that prevent you from following the medication regimen?
Storage	Where are your medications stored at home?
	How long do you keep medications in the home?
	Can you show me any medications you have on hand?

INDEX

Note: Page numbers followed by *f* indicate figures.

A
Accident reports, 19
Age considerations
    for injection administration, 39
    for medication administration, 31–32
    for starting intravenous fusion, 45
Ampule, 6, 7*f*, 23*f*–24*f*
Auditory canal, 42*f*

B
Bolus IV medication, 55*f*–56*f*

C
Capsule, features of, 63
Cartridges, prefilled, 7
Central venous access device, 50
Children
    ear drops instillation in, 17*f*
    medication administration to, 4
    starting intravenous fusion for, 45
Continuous infusion, 13
Creams, 14, 16

D
Deltoid muscle site, 11
Diabetic patients, 8, 28
Diazepam (Valium), 7
Dorsogluteal site, 11
Dressing. *See* IV dressing
Drugs. *See* Medication(s)

E
Ear drops
    instillation of, 16
    nursing care guidelines for, 17*f*
Ear irrigations
    administration of, 41*f*–42*f*
    purpose of, 16
Elixir, features of, 63
Enteral feeding tube, 5
Enteric-coated tablets, 3
Extended release medication, 63
Eyedrops
    instillation of, 14
    procedure, 15*f*
Eye irrigation
    administration of, 40*f*–41*f*
    purpose of, 15–16
Eye medication disks, 16

H
Heparin
    administration of, 9
    lock, 60–61, 62*f*
Home care considerations
    for injection administration, 36
    for medication administration, 32

I
Inhalation, medication administration by, 17–18, 63

Injection(s). *See also specific types*
    intradermal, 8
    medication administration by, 6–7
    subcutaneous, 8–9
Injection site
    cleaning, 35*f*
    identifying landmarks for, 38*f*
Insulin administration, 8, 9, 27*f*–28*f*
Intermittent intravenous infusion, 13, 52
Intermittent venous access device, 13
Intradermal injections/route
    administration of, 8, 32*f*–33*f*
    angle of insertion for, 11*f*
Intramuscular injections/route
    administration of, 37*f*–39*f*
    angle of insertion for, 11*f*
    medication administration through, 9
    procedure, 11
    reducing discomfort in, 12
    sites for, 9, 10*f*, 11
    Z-track technique for, 11–12
Intravenous fusion/site
    intermittent, 13, 52
    monitoring, 48*f*–49*f*
    starting, 42*f*–45*f*
Intravenous lock, 13, 60–61, 62*f*
Intravenous route, 12–13
Inunction, 14
IV catheter, disconnecting tubing from, 52*f*
IV dressing, changing, 49*f*–51*f*
IV medications, bolus, 55*f*–56*f*
IV solution and tubing
    adding medication to, 53*f*–54*f*
    changing, 46*f*–47*f*

K
Kardex, 29, 30*f*

L
Liniment, features of, 63
Lotions, features of, 14, 63
Lozenge, features of, 63

M
Medication(s)
    abuse and, 19, 21–22
    adding, 53*f*–54*f*
    disguising objectionable taste of, 4
    errors, 18–19
    extended release, 63
    factors to assess, 64
    incompatibility issues, 7
    injecting, 33*f*, 36*f*, 56*f*, 59*f*
    mixing, 7*f*, 8
    omitted, 18
    patient's refusal to, 18
    powdered, 8
    preparations, 63
    sublingual, 5
    through heparin or intravenous lock, 60–61, 62*f*
Medication administration
    documenting, 18–19
    by inhalation, 17–18, 63
    by injection, 6–7
    intradermal route, 8, 32*f*–33*f*
    intramuscular route, 9–12, 37*f*–39*f*

intravenous route, 12–13
    nursing responsibilities for, 4
    oral, 3–4, 29*f*–32*f*, 63
    parenteral route, 5–6, 63
    by piggyback pump, 13, 57–58, 59*f*
    routes for, 63
    subcutaneous route, 8–9, 34*f*–36*f*
    techniques, 4–5
    topical application, 13–17
Medication record
    example of, 20–21
    medication errors and, 18
Medication removal
    from an ampule, 23–24
    from a vial, 25–26
Metered-dose inhaler (MDI), 18
Miniinfusion pump, 57–58, 59*f*

N
Narcotics, 3
Nebulization, 18
Needleless system, 6*f*
Needles
    inserting, 33*f*, 35*f*
    parts of, 6*f*
    syringes and, 5
    withdrawing, 36*f*
Nose drops, 16, 18
Nursing care guidelines
    for instilling ear drops, 17*f*
    for instilling eyedrops, 15*f*
    for instilling nose drops, 18
    for transdermal patches, 14

O
Oils, 14
Ointments, 14, 15, 63
Older adults
    ear drops instillation in, 17*f*
    medication administration to, 4–5
    starting intravenous fusion for, 45
Oral medications/route, 3–4, 29*f*–32*f*, 63

P
Parenteral medications/route
    administration of, 5
    description of, 63
    needleless system and, 6
    needles and syringes and, 5–6
Patients
    checking identity of, 30, 31*f*
    guidelines for, 21–22
    refusal to drugs, 18
    response to infusion, recording, 47*f*
Piggyback delivery system, 13, 57–58, 59*f*
Pill, features of, 63
Powdered medications, reconstituting, 8
Powders, features of, 14, 63
Prefilled cartridges, 7
Primary line capping, 52*f*
Procedures
    adding bolus IV medication, 55–56
    adding medication to IV solution, 53–54
    capping a primary line, 52
    changing an IV dressing, 49–51
    changing IV solution and tubing, 46–47
    ear irrigation administration, 41–42
    eye irrigation administration, 40–41